Body in Balar

Your Guide to Taming Inflammation

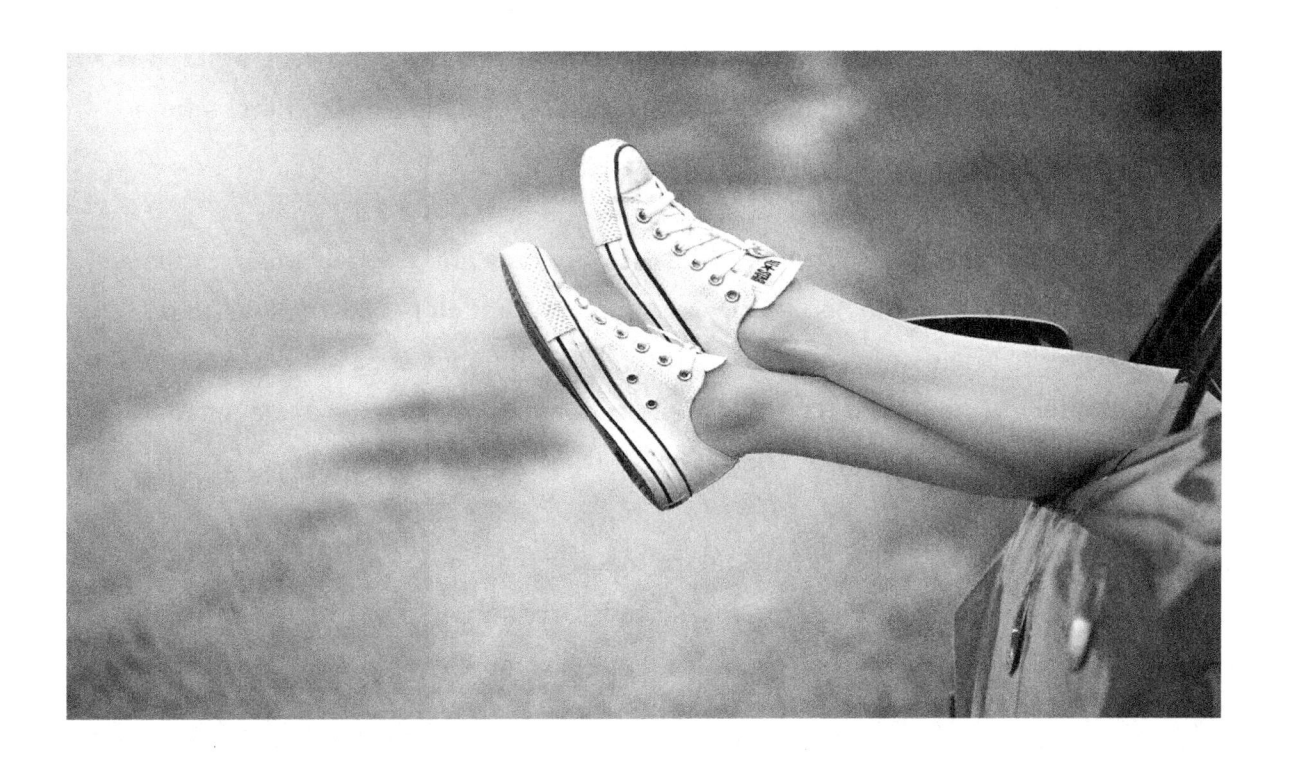

Margaret K. Lapham

Copyright © Margaret K. Lapham, 2024

All rights reserved. No part of this publication may be reproduced, distributed, or transmitted in any form or by any means, including photocopying, recording, or other electronic or mechanical methods, without the prior written permission of the publisher, except in the case of brief quotations embodied in critical reviews and certain other noncommercial uses permitted by copyright law.

Disclaimer Page

This book is presented as is, without warranty of any kind, either express or implied, including, but not limited to, the implied warranties of merchantability, fitness for a particular purpose, or non-infringement.

The author has made every effort to ensure the accuracy and completeness of the information contained in this book. However, the information is provided without warranty, either express or implied. The author and publisher shall have neither liability nor responsibility to any person or entity with respect to any loss or damages arising from the information contained in this book.

This book is not intended as a substitute for the medical advice of physicians or other healthcare professionals. The reader should regularly consult a physician in matters relating to their health and particularly with respect to any symptoms that may require diagnosis or medical attention.

The views expressed in this book are solely those of the author and do not necessarily reflect the views of the publisher or any other affiliated organizations.

Any trademarks, service marks, product names, or named features are assumed to be the property of their respective owners and are used only for reference. There is no implied endorsement if these terms are used in this book.

Contents

UNDERSTANDING INFLAMMATION..4
   Inflammation's Effect on General Health..6
   Historical perspective...8
   Contemporary methods..10

1. THE DUAL NATURE OF INFLAMMATION..13
   Inflammation as a Defender...13
   Why Acute Inflammation Guards Against Us..................................15
   Persistent Inflammation...17
   Regaining Balance..19
   The Effect of Inflammation on Hormones.......................................21

2. STRESS REDUCTION...23
   The Modern Stress Epidemic..23
   Practical Stress-Reduction Methods...25
   Recognizing When to Seek Professional Help...............................28
   Integrated Medical Methods..31
   Takeaways for Putting Stress Management Strategies Into Practice............32

3. NUTRITION..35
   Feeding Your Microbiome...35
   Curcumin with Anti-Inflammatory Herbs...39
      The Top 10 Spices to Reduce Inflammation..............................39
   How to Incorporate Anti-Inflammatory Seasonings into Your Diet..........42
   How to Recognize Inflammatory Foods..44
   How to Gradually Cut Out Inflammatory Foods..............................46
   Exploring Anti-Inflammatory Diets...48
      Mediterranean Diet...48
      DASH Diet..49
      Paleo Diet...49
      Whole30 Diet..49
   The Autoimmune Protocol (AIP)..50
   Plant-Based Eating..54
   Getting Rid of Gluten...56
   The Benefits of Food Journaling...57
   Making the First Dietary Adjustments...60

4. TARGETED SUPPLEMENTATION...63
   Essential Anti-Inflammatory Supplements......................................63
   The Link Between Prebiotics and Probiotics..................................66

    Natural Probiotic Sources...68
    Tailored Supplements...71
5. MINDFUL ALCOHOL CONSUMPTION...73
    Alcohol's Effects..73
    Moderate Alcohol Use...74
    Advantages of Cutting Back on Drinking...75
    Recognizing Problematic Drinking...77
    The Effects of Excess Alcohol on Health...79
    Alcohol-Free Substitutes...81
6. RESTORATIVE SLEEP...84
    The Ideal Sleeping Time...85
    Resolving Sleep Deficit...86
    Lack of sleep and inflammation..87
    Fostering Restful Sleep Practices..88
    Your Sleep Improvement Toolkit..89
    When to Speak with a Sleep Expert..91
    Options for Sleep Disorder Treatment...92
7. BALANCED PHYSICAL ACTIVITY..96
    Using Exercise as a Tool to Reduce Inflammation...96
    Deciding on the Ideal Balance for Exercise..98
    Low-impact, home-based exercises..100
    Special Considerations for Exercise..102
    Optimizing Exercise's Effects...104
8. HOLISTIC SELF-CARE...110
    Inflammation of the System and Dental Health..111
    Therapeutic Massage Benefits..112
    Finding Toxins in the Environment..114
    Skin Health and Protection...116
    Inflammatory Effects of Smoking...117
    Giving Up Smoking...118
    Activities & Hobbies that Reduce Stress..120
Conclusion..124

UNDERSTANDING INFLAMMATION

Think of your body as a stronghold that is always on the lookout for intruders and potential dangers. When danger hits, inflammation acts as your body's army, rushing to your defense. It's a normal, necessary process that aids in the defense and restoration of your body. However, like with many things, excess of a positive attribute may have negative effects.

Fundamentally, inflammation is the reaction of your immune system to injury. Your body reacts to injuries such as paper cuts, sprained ankles, and viruses by mobilizing resources to heal the wound. Your body may experience redness, swelling, heat, and perhaps discomfort throughout this process—all indications that it is working hard!

Acute vs Chronic Inflammation

Consider acute inflammation to be your body's "good cop" " After being called upon, it arrives promptly, gets the job done, and leaves after the issue is over. This is the swelling you get when you get a cold or cut your toe. It's really important for healing, but it's transient, usually lasting a few days to a few weeks.

When you cut your finger, for instance:
1. The nearby blood vessels enlarge, supplying extra blood to the region.
2. White blood cells infiltrate the area to combat any possible illnesses.
3. A build-up of fluid results in swelling, which aids in immobilizing the region.
4. After the danger is eliminated, the healing process is finished and the inflammation goes down.

Conversely, chronic inflammation is comparable to an overly vigilant security guard who never leaves the office. This kind of inflammation is low-grade and chronic, and it may linger for many months or even years. Contrary to its acute cousin, chronic inflammation often goes unnoticed and gradually harms your health.

Many things might set off this troublemaker, including:
- Injuries or illnesses left untreated

- Immune system conditions
- Being around poisons
- Prolonged stress
- Unhealthy food and lifestyle choices

Numerous health problems have been linked to chronic inflammation, including diabetes, heart disease, cancer, and neurological diseases. It's similar to a slow-burning fire within your body that may go out of control and do major harm.

Let's now examine more closely the underlying processes of inflammation;

Your body issues alarm signals when it senses a hazard, whether it is an injury, an illness, or an irritation. These are substances known as chemokines and cytokines. Consider them the body's equivalent of a fire alarm, warning other cells in the vicinity that something is wrong. The impacted area's blood vessels widen in reaction to these warning messages. This is analogous to widening a highway's lanes to accommodate more vehicles. Here, the "traffic" is more blood flowing, and more immune cells are traveling with it. White blood cells show up, especially macrophages and neutrophils. These are the security detail and cleaning staff all bundled into one for your body. They take up and eliminate dangerous infections, broken cells, and detritus. Blood arteries become more porous during the inflammatory reaction, which permits fluid and proteins to seep into the surrounding tissues. This is the reason for the edema or swelling that we connect with inflammation. It resembles putting a cushion of protection around the wounded region. Once the immediate danger has been neutralized, another cell type takes control. Among them are fibroblasts, which produce collagen and other healing-related proteins and aid in tissue repair. Anti-inflammatory mechanisms take over in acute inflammation after the danger has been eliminated and healing has begun. Your body is telling you, "Okay, team, great job." It's time to go and pack.

But in cases of chronic inflammation, this instruction to stand down is either ignored or misunderstood. Even in the absence of an obvious danger, the inflammatory reaction persists.

We can better comprehend the intricacy of our body's defensive systems and the significance of maintaining a balanced inflammatory response when we have a better understanding of these processes. We'll examine how different lifestyle choices might affect these processes in the next chapters, as well as strategies for promoting healthy inflammation.

Inflammation is an essential component of our body's healing process; it is not the enemy. The human objective is to avoid low-grade, chronic inflammation that might eventually compromise human health while simultaneously promoting acute inflammation when it is required.

Inflammation's Effect on General Health

We now know that inflammation has two drawbacks. Even while it's necessary for recovery and defense against dangers, when it goes wrong, our health may suffer greatly. Think of inflammation as a bodily fire. An uncontrolled fire may wreak havoc yet a managed fire can cook your meal and keep you warm. This is exactly how our bodies deal with chronic inflammation.

When inflammation progresses to a chronic state, it spreads throughout the body. Rather, it embeds itself in our systems, interfering with everything from our heart to our brain. Over time, this systemic inflammation may harm our systems covertly and often without our knowledge. It works like a cunning saboteur, gradually destroying our health from the inside out.

The connection between chronic inflammation and chronic illnesses is one of the most important ways that chronic inflammation affects human health. Inflammation is at the root of a lot of the health problems that afflict contemporary society. For example, heart disease is not just related to cholesterol. Atherosclerosis, or the accumulation of plaque in our arteries, is mostly influenced by inflammation. It seems like inflammation is continually prodding our blood vessel walls, creating damage that eventually results in the buildup of fatty deposits.

Heart disease is not the end of the narrative, however. Numerous medical disorders have been linked to chronic inflammation. For example, there is a close relationship between inflammation and diabetes. Inflammatory substances may impede insulin signaling and cause insulin resistance, which is a defining feature of type 2 diabetes. It seems as if the locks that insulin utilizes to get glucose into our cells are being jammed by inflammation.

The consequences of persistent inflammation might even affect our mental wellness. Intriguing connections have been discovered by researchers between anxiety and mental health issues including depression and anxiety. Our brain chemistry seems to be impacted by the inflammatory process, which may have an impact on our mood and cognitive abilities. This link contributes to the understanding of why mood problems are often experienced by those with long-term inflammatory illnesses.

The connection between inflammation and aging is perhaps one of the most intriguing features of inflammation. Scientists refer to this process of increased inflammatory responses in our bodies as "inflammaging." Not only is this age-related rise in inflammation a consequence of becoming older, but it also actively promotes aging.

Imagine inflammatory responses as a slow-burning fire that eventually destroys our body's systems. It may accelerate the deterioration of collagen, causing wrinkles and loose skin. It could be a factor in the age-related decline of strength and muscular mass. Since persistent inflammation has been connected to a higher risk of neurodegenerative illnesses like Alzheimer's, even our cognitive function may be negatively impacted.

The good news is that we now have strong tools to safeguard our health as a result of our growing knowledge of the role inflammation plays in aging and illness. We may be able to slow down the aging process and lower our chance of developing chronic illnesses by managing inflammation. It functions similarly to a fire extinguisher for a smoldering, flaming fire.

This is where lifestyle decisions are relevant. Our lifestyle choices, including what we eat, how much we walk, how well we sleep, and how we handle stress, all have a significant impact on internal inflammation. We may encourage a balanced inflammatory response by making well-informed decisions, which will support our body's natural healing processes without allowing inflammation to spiral out of control.

We'll look at doable tactics to control inflammation and promote general well-being. You'll find a multitude of solutions to assist you in managing your inflammatory fire, ranging from stress-reduction methods to anti-inflammatory meals. Recall that the objective is not to eradicate inflammation, since it would be unfeasible and unwelcome. Rather, our goal is to balance, bolstering our body's natural defenses while avoiding low-grade, chronic inflammation that over time might compromise our health.

Historical perspective

The history of inflammatory research is an intriguing one, reflecting how our knowledge of the human body has changed throughout time. This is a story of how curiosity, ground-breaking discoveries, and paradigm changes have influenced contemporary medicine.

The primary indicators of inflammation—redness, heat, swelling, and pain—were first noticed by astute observers in ancient civilizations thousands of years ago, which is when our investigation into inflammation got its start. In the first century AD, the Roman encyclopedist Celsus provided a formal description of these indicators, setting the stage for further research. It's amazing to consider that these first findings, conducted before the invention of microscopes or contemporary technologies, nonetheless serve as the cornerstone of our knowledge today.

For generations, the main perception of inflammation was that it was a bad process. Bloodletting was often employed to "draw out" inflammation; it was a technique that lasted long into the 19th century. Even though we now understand that this approach was more detrimental than beneficial, it nevertheless represents the widespread notion that inflammation should be eradicated from the body at all costs.

Understanding inflammation was revolutionized in the 19th century. With the development of the microscope, scientists were able to see cellular activities for the first time, opening up a whole new universe. Loss of function was the fifth cardinal sign that Rudolf Virchow, who is sometimes referred to as the "father of modern pathology," added to Celsus's list around this time. Thanks in part to Virchow's work, attention has shifted from outward manifestations of inflammation to the underlying molecular mechanisms.

The 20th century saw further advancements in our knowledge of inflammation. An important turning point was Elie Metchnikoff's discovery of phagocytes in the late 1800s. Metchnikoff saw cells consuming foreign objects, a process that is today understood to be essential for the inflammatory response. He was awarded the Nobel Prize for this finding, which also helped us to comprehend the immune system's function in inflammation today.

Another major development in our knowledge of inflammation occurred in the middle of the 20th century. Scientists started identifying chemicals such as prostaglandins, bradykinin, and histamine that act as chemical mediators of inflammation. Anti-inflammatory medications, such as corticosteroids and non-steroidal anti-inflammatory Drugs (NSAIDs), were developed as a result of this understanding and are now mainstays of contemporary medicine.

However, the second half of the 20th century saw possibly the most significant change in our knowledge of inflammation, and this trend continues today. Scholars began to acknowledge inflammation not alone as a reaction to harm or infection, but also as a pivotal element in an extensive array of persistent illnesses. New paths for the diagnosis and surveillance of inflammatory disorders were made possible by the identification of inflammatory markers such as C-reactive protein.

Research on the role of inflammation in illnesses ranging from cancer and neurodegenerative disorders to diabetes and heart disease has exploded in the last few decades. Gerontology's "inflammaging" theory—which refers to low-grade, chronic inflammation that tends to worsen with aging—has become a major field of research.

Inflammation is now understood to be a complicated, multifaceted process that may have both positive and negative effects. The emphasis now is on modulating inflammation for optimum health rather than just suppressing it. For example, studies on the gut microbiome are uncovering intriguing links between systemic inflammation, gut flora, and our nutrition.

There is still much to learn about inflammation as we stand on the brink of fresh discoveries. Novel approaches to studying inflammation, such as gene editing and artificial intelligence, have great potential. Who knows what new findings may be made?

This lengthy history of studying inflammation serves as a reminder that centuries of observation, investigation, and discovery have led to the present state of our knowledge. It's a monument to human curiosity and tenacity, and it offers a strong starting point for the useful tactics we'll cover in this book. We are expanding on this extensive history of scientific investigation as we investigate strategies to control inflammation in our day-to-day lives, transforming historical findings and state-of-the-art research into doable actions for improved health.

Contemporary methods

Our strategy for controlling inflammation has changed significantly in the last several years. A more sophisticated, comprehensive approach that acknowledges the multifaceted function inflammation plays in our bodies has replaced the one-size-fits-all method of merely decreasing inflammation. This change reflects our increasing realization that inflammation is not an adversary to be defeated, but rather a delicate balancing act.

Precision and customization are key components of contemporary inflammation control. We now know that an individualized strategy is necessary for successful inflammation management and that what works for one person may not work for another. It's similar to leading an orchestra in that every instrument has a certain function to perform, and when they all work together harmoniously, beautiful health is the outcome.

Nutrition is a key component in contemporary inflammation control. We now understand that food provides our bodies with information in addition to fuel. While certain meals might help reduce inflammation, others can increase it. For example, the Mediterranean diet's anti-inflammatory qualities have come to light. This diet, which is high in fruits, vegetables, whole grains, and healthy fats like olive oil, has been shown to lower the body's inflammatory indicators. It seems as if we are adjusting our inflammatory response with our forks.

However, timing is just as important as content when it comes to eating. One possible tactic for controlling inflammation is intermittent fasting. Our ability to reset our inflammatory responses could be achieved by allowing our digestive system frequent rests. It's similar to restarting the inflammatory processes in our bodies.

In addition to its extensive list of health advantages, exercise is also understood to be an effective strategy for reducing inflammation. It has been shown that regular, moderate exercise offers anti-inflammatory benefits. It's similar to bringing your immune system to the gym to work on improving its response to inflammatory stimuli. Nonetheless, the crucial term in this context is moderate - excessive exercise may exacerbate inflammation, highlighting the need to maintain equilibrium in our strategy.

Modern inflammation control has also placed a strong emphasis on stress management. Deep breathing exercises, yoga, and mindfulness meditation are all important additions to our anti-inflammatory toolbox since chronic stress may exacerbate inflammation. By encouraging the parasympathetic nervous system to become active, these techniques may help reduce excessive inflammatory reactions by putting the body in "rest and digest" mode.

Sleep, which was previously undervalued, is now shown to be essential for reducing inflammation. Our bodies carry out critical maintenance tasks when we sleep, including controlling inflammatory processes. Making proper sleep hygiene a priority is similar to allowing our bodies the time off to adjust their inflammatory responses.

A more focused strategy is emerging in the supplement industry. There's a rising focus on tailored supplementing based on individual requirements rather than general suggestions. Probiotics, curcumin, and omega-3 fatty acids are a few supplements that have shown potential in the treatment of inflammation.

About probiotics, the gut microbiota is now a key component of contemporary inflammation control. It is now established that the billions of bacteria that reside in our digestive tract are essential for controlling inflammation throughout the body. Anti-inflammatory diets now include tactics to maintain a healthy gut flora, such as eating fermented foods and avoiding needless antibiotic use.

In the field of medicine, inflammatory disorders are being treated using more advanced methods. Biologics are a class of pharmaceuticals that target certain immune system components and have completely changed how many inflammatory and autoimmune disorders are treated. It's similar to having medical-grade missiles that can accurately target harmful inflammatory processes while sparing healthy ones.

The potential of cannabinoids, especially CBD, to reduce inflammation is also gaining attention. Although studies are still in their early phases, preliminary findings indicate that these substances may provide novel approaches to the management of inflammation.

The area of nutritional genomics is one of the most fascinating ones, maybe. This new field of study examines how our unique genetic make-up affects how we react to various nutrients and meals. We could eventually be able to design customized anti-inflammatory diets according to our genetic profiles.

As time goes on, prevention becomes more and more important than merely therapy. Through a proactive lifestyle and an awareness of our risk factors, we may be able to stop chronic inflammation before it starts.

It is not possible to treat inflammation today with miracle cures or fast remedies. Rather, the goal is to establish a state in our bodies where inflammation may function when necessary without becoming excessive. It's a holistic approach that takes into account every facet of our lives, including our thoughts, feelings, and physical and nutritional habits.

1. THE DUAL NATURE OF INFLAMMATION

Inflammation as a Defender

Our bodies are amazing machines, equipped with a complex defense and repair mechanism that activates at the first indication of danger. The ability of our biology to cure itself is a monument to its wisdom, developed over millions of years of evolution. Inflammation, our body's first line of defense against damage and infection, is at the center of this process.

Let's say you just scraped your knee on the pavement. In a few seconds, your body initiates an intricate sequence of actions intended to safeguard you against injury and initiate the recuperation process. This is the function of acute inflammation, which is an essential tool in your body's self-healing repertoire.

Acute inflammation is a well-coordinated sequence of events, each of which is essential to the preservation and repair of your body.

The first phase starts almost right away after an injury. The afflicted area's blood arteries widen, bringing more blood to the location. It seems like your body is widening all road lanes to expedite the arrival of emergency personnel. An injury's surrounding redness and warmth are the result of increased blood flow.

The stage of vascular permeability follows. Small blood artery walls become more porous, enabling the passage of fluid and proteins into the surrounding tissues. This results in swelling, or edema, which is not only painful but also has a vital function. While the fluid contains vital cells and chemicals required for healing, the swelling aids in immobilizing the region and shielding it from more harm.

Your body is also enlisting the help of its cellular defenses at this time. Neutrophils, for instance, are among the first white blood cells to reach the scene. Similar to your immune system's initial responders, these cells are prepared to take up and eliminate any dangerous germs that may have gotten into the wound.

Other subsets of white blood cells, such as macrophages, trail closely after neutrophils. In addition to carrying out the cleansing, these cells also emit signaling chemicals that aid in coordinating the subsequent phases of healing.

Your body starts the process of repairing damaged tissue at the next stage if the injury is more serious. Fibroblasts, which are specialized cells, proliferate and produce collagen and other proteins that aid in the healing process of the injured tissue. It functions similarly to your body's construction staff, repairing any damage.

Eventually, the inflammatory response starts to lessen as healing advances. Redness disappears, swelling decreases, and your body gradually reverts to its original form. This is an important resolution step, your body's way of telling you, "Mission accomplished."

An ensemble of molecular characteristics is crucial in directing the inflammatory response throughout this phase. Each of these important inflammatory mediators has a distinct role to perform, much like the directors and producers of your body's healing production.

Mostly secreted by mast cells, histamine is often one of the first mediators to be released. It opens up blood vessels and increases their permeability, which initiates the inflammatory reaction. The first redness and swelling you see in an inflammatory region are caused by histamine.

Another significant class of mediators is prostaglandins. Similar to your body's multifunctional instruments, they aid in increasing blood flow, eliciting pain signals that shield the afflicted region, and, when necessary, assisting in the resolution of inflammation.

The specialists in communication in the inflammatory process are called cytokines. As messengers, these proteins mobilize more immune cells, initiate the synthesis of acute-phase proteins, and facilitate the inflammatory response as a whole. Tumor necrosis factor (TNF) and interleukin-1 (IL-1) are two examples of cytokines that have pro-inflammatory properties, while interleukin-10 (IL-10) has an anti-inflammatory impact.

A system made up of complement proteins aids in the removal of infections from the body via phagocytic cells and antibodies. They act as your immune system's bouncers, marking trespassers for elimination.

Finally, chemokines are the traffic controllers of inflammation. Your body's protectors reach the area of inflammation precisely because of these tiny proteins, which direct white blood cells there.

Gaining knowledge about these phases and inflammatory mediators helps us better appreciate how intricate and effective our body's self-healing mechanism is. It's a well-tuned mechanism that can react to many different types of injuries and dangers. We'll look at what occurs when this system malfunctions and causes chronic inflammation in the next sections, as well as how we may encourage our body's natural healing processes with certain lifestyle modifications and treatments.

Why Acute Inflammation Guards Against Us

When problems arise, acute inflammation acts as your body's superhero, coming to your rescue. It is an essential component of our immune system that helps us respond quickly and effectively to infections, wounds, and other health risks. Acute inflammation is not a sign of trouble; rather, it is an indication that everything in your body is functioning as it should.

Consider your body to be a stronghold. Acute inflammation may be thought of as the first responder, the alarm system, and the repair team together. When pathogens, viruses, or physical wounds break the walls, inflammation mobilizes the defenses, neutralizes the danger, and starts the healing process.

The main way that acute inflammation keeps us safe is by keeping dangerous stimuli in check and getting rid of them. For instance, inflammation aids in the separation of the foreign item and any germs it may contain when you acquire a splinter. Immune cells are drawn to the location by the swelling and increased blood flow, where they are prepared to fight off any possible infection.

Another important factor in the healing process is inflammation. Inflammatory mediators set off a series of processes after an injury that eventually results in tissue healing. Wounds would heal much more slowly without this inflammatory response, making us more susceptible to infection and further harm.

Let's examine a few commonplace situations when acute inflammation saves the day:

You may have a runny nose, sore throat, and overall discomfort when you have a cold. In reality, these symptoms are indicators that the inflammatory reaction in your body is trying to combat the viral infection. Your body is signaled to relax and redirect its resources towards the immunological response by the inflammation, which also aids in capturing and eradicating the virus.

You've seen inflammation in action if you've ever twisted your ankle. The ensuing swelling aids in immobilizing the joint and halting more damage. Meanwhile, faster healing occurs because of increased blood flow, which supplies healing elements to the location.

A paper cut, for example, may cause an inflammatory reaction. Your body will try to heal the wound and stop an infection, which may cause the region to become red and swollen. This localized inflammation is a perfect illustration of how your body may react appropriately to a danger.

Part of the reason you experience slight discomfort after a good exercise is acute inflammation. Over time, your strength and endurance will increase as a result of your body using this inflammatory reaction as a signal to strengthen and heal the strained muscles.

White blood cells are the unsung heroes of our immune system; they are at the center of the inflammatory response. These cells perform several functions that keep us safe and aid in our recovery.

When inflammation occurs, neutrophils are often the first white blood cells to reach the area. They operate as your immune system's initial responders, moving quickly to engulf and eliminate dangerous microorganisms. Additionally, the substances released by neutrophils attract other immune cells to the region, intensifying the inflammatory response.

Macrophages are the immune system's cleanup team. They are more persistent than neutrophils, although they come a little later. In addition to consuming infections and cellular waste, macrophages are essential for the healing of wounds. They exude growth factors, which promote the restoration of blood vessels and injured tissues.

Your immune system's special troops are T-cells and B-cells. They are more important for adaptive immunity, but they also have an impact on the inflammatory response. To coordinate the immune response, T-cells may target infected cells directly and produce cytokines. Antibodies produced by B-cells mark infections so that other immune cells may destroy them.

Despite being less common than other white blood cells, eosinophils and basophils are crucial for certain inflammatory reactions, especially those involving allergies and parasite infections.

This system is beautiful because it can react appropriately to many dangers. A more severe illness might cause a more extensive inflammatory response, but a little paper cut might only need a limited, localized response.

It's crucial to keep in mind that, despite the common perception of inflammation as something bad, acute inflammation is an essential and beneficial activity. It's a signal that your body is using a lot of energy to defend and restore you. Only when inflammation becomes severe or chronic—as we'll discuss in the next sections—do problems occur.

Through comprehension and appreciation of the defensive function of acute inflammation, we may enhance our body's inherent healing mechanisms. We'll talk about how lifestyle decisions may support a healthy inflammatory response in the next chapters so that this important process continues to support rather than compromise our health.

Persistent Inflammation

Indications and Markers of Prolonged Inflammation

It's common to compare chronic inflammation to a quiet fire that burns within the body. Chronic inflammation may be modest and long-lasting, in contrast to acute inflammation, which is usually evident and transient. It may slowly erode your health, much like a slow-burning fire if ignored.

Certain visual indicators of persistent inflammation act as outside cues to the underlying bodily processes that are taking place:

Persistent joint swelling is a highly identifiable indicator of chronic inflammation, especially in disorders such as rheumatoid arthritis. Affected joints may feel warm to the touch and seem bigger than usual.

Skin Problems: There are many ways that chronic inflammation may show up on the skin. Disorders like psoriasis, which is characterized by red, scaly patches, or chronic acne may indicate the presence of underlying inflammation. Some folks may also have hives or rashes that don't seem to go away.

Puffiness: Persistent inflammation may be indicated by general puffiness, particularly in the face or around the eyes. Fluid retention, a typical inflammatory reaction, is often to blame for this.

Redness: Persistent redness in the afflicted regions might be a symptom of chronic inflammation. This might be especially apparent on the face, such as in cases of rosacea.

Nonetheless, a lot of chronic inflammatory signs are imperceptible to the unaided eye. The following "invisible" symptoms may have an equal negative effect on your quality of life:

Fatigue: One of the most prevalent signs of chronic inflammation is a persistent weariness that doesn't go away with rest. It seems like your body is engaged in combat all the time, depleting your vitality.

Mood Shifts: Anxiety and despair are two mood disorders that have been connected to chronic inflammation. You may get irritable, have inexplicable mood fluctuations, or have a chronically depressed mood.

Brain Fog: Chronic inflammation is often associated with a sensation of mental cloudiness or trouble focusing, which is sometimes referred to as "brain fog."

Digestive Problems: Bloating, constipation, or diarrhea are just a few of the symptoms that may arise from chronic inflammation of the digestive tract.

Chronic Pain: Chronic inflammation is often indicated by persistent, widespread pain that is not related to a particular injury.

Sleep disturbances: Prolonged inflammation may be a contributing factor in trouble getting to sleep or staying asleep.

Weight Changes: Chronic inflammation may be the cause of unexplained weight gain or resistance to weight reduction.

Regaining Balance

Knowing the importance of anti-inflammatory lifestyle choices is like finding a master key that opens many doors to wellness on our path to greater health. These options provide a comprehensive approach to inflammation treatment that may significantly improve your entire quality of life, rather than merely treating a particular health issue.

Consider your body as an instrument with precise tuning. To reach maximum health, we must nurture our bodies in the same way that a musician must take care of their instrument to make beautiful music. We maintain the harmony of our body 'instrument' with everyday routines that are anti-inflammatory.

A holistic approach acknowledges the interdependence of our body's systems. Affected areas of our bodies always have an impact on the whole body. Because of this interdependence, when we make decisions that lower inflammation, we're not just treating one symptom or illness; rather, we're fostering general health and vitality.

For instance, eating anti-inflammatory foods may help your mood, increase your energy, and even improve the look of your skin in addition to your digestive system. Similarly, practicing yoga or meditation to manage your stress may not only help you relax mentally but also lower inflammation in your body, which may help with joint pain or heart health.

Using a comprehensive approach gives us the ability to take charge of our health. By making everyday decisions and developing healthy habits, we may actively contribute to our wellness rather than just depending on drugs to treat symptoms.

Living an anti-inflammatory lifestyle has several advantages beyond just reducing inflammation right away. It's a long-term investment that will pay off in terms of improved health.

You may see short-term increases in your mood, energy, and overall wellness. However, the true magic occurs gradually.

1. Lowering your chance of developing long-term conditions including diabetes, heart disease, and certain types of cancer.
2. Helping you age healthily and maybe living a longer life.
3. Lowering the risk of neurodegenerative illnesses and enhancing cognitive performance.
4. Strengthening your body's innate capacity to recover from diseases or injuries.
5. Increasing your resistance to illnesses by strengthening your immune system.

It compares to starting a garden. Every decision you make to reduce inflammation is a seed. These seeds develop into a colorful, health-giving garden that feeds you for years to come with regular attention and patience.

The Effect of Inflammation on Hormones

The production and regulation of hormones that govern different physiological processes is the responsibility of the endocrine system, which is significantly impacted by inflammation. Inflammation throws off the delicate balance between hormone synthesis and reception, altering our bodies' normal functioning in profound ways.

Inflammation modifies the synthesis of hormones, which affects hormone levels and activity. Reproductive function, growth and development, and metabolism are all impacted in turn by this. For instance, increased cortisol production from inflammation may cause mood swings, weight gain, and insulin resistance.

Hormone receptor sensitivity is impacted by inflammation as well, changing how sensitive they are to hormones. This further messes with the control of hormones, which modifies the way cells react to hormone signals. Wide-ranging effects of inflammation on hormone receptors include modifications to mood control, energy metabolism, and reproductive function.

Inflammation significantly affects the HPA axis and cortisol. When there is inflammation, the HPA axis is triggered, which increases the production of cortisol. Insulin resistance, mood swings, and weight gain are just a few of the terrible consequences that may result from persistently high cortisol levels. Inflammation also affects thyroid hormones, which alters energy levels and metabolism.

Inflammation also affects sex hormones, such as testosterone and estrogen. This may result in changes in mood, general health, and reproductive function. Lastly, inflammation has a role in insulin resistance by impeding the uptake of glucose into cells and altering the control of blood sugar. We can better comprehend the significance of managing inflammation to enhance general health and well-being by knowing how it affects hormone control.

We looked at the dual nature of inflammation in this chapter, emphasizing how important it is to our body's defense against damage and infection as well as how it can be harmful if left unchecked. We spoke about how inflammation alters the endocrine system, causing disruptions to hormone synthesis and reception as well as modifications to energy levels, metabolism, and reproductive function. We also looked at how inflammation affected cortisol, thyroid, sex, and insulin hormones, among other hormones.

Important lessons learned:

- Although inflammation is a normal reaction, when it persists over time, it may be dangerous.
- Hormone balance may be upset by chronic inflammation, which can alter metabolism, energy levels, and reproductive function.
- Inflammation affects some hormones, such as insulin, sex hormones, thyroid hormones, and cortisol.

2. STRESS REDUCTION

The Modern Stress Epidemic

Millions of people worldwide suffer from stress, which has become an omnipresent aspect of contemporary life. The figures are concerning. The American Psychological Association reports that moderate to high levels of stress are experienced by 75% of individuals. According to the World Health Organization, the cost of stress-related disorders to the worldwide economy is $300 billion yearly, making this pandemic of stress expensive. Stress is a major public health concern since it causes mental health problems in 1 in 5 persons.

Stress levels are growing globally, according to global stress trends, with some nations having greater stress levels than others. The nations that are under the most stress include China, South Africa, Nigeria, India, and the United States. In terms of demographics, young people (18–25) report greater levels of stress than older ones, while women report higher levels than males. In addition, stress levels are greater in low-income persons than in high-income ones.

Chronic stress is exacerbated by several factors in modern living. It's difficult to unplug and unwind when faced with technology and continuous connectedness, which induces a state of continual awareness. Problems with work-life balance include lengthy work hours, transportation, and the expectation to be accessible at all times, which make it difficult to distinguish between work and personal life. Stress levels might rise due to information overload from news, social media, and other information sources. If ignored, these elements combine to produce a perfect storm of stress that may have detrimental effects on one's physical and emotional well-being.

Our natural, evolutionary-preserved stress response aids in our ability to respond to dangers and obstacles. Alternatively referred to as the fight-or-flight response, it primes our systems to either engage the danger or escape it. Our body is hardwired with this reaction, which has its origins in the survival tactics of our ancestors.

Stress was essential to our ancestors' survival from an evolutionary standpoint. The stress reaction made it possible for them to respond swiftly and improve their chances of survival when they were threatened by a predator or another threat. Even though a lot has changed in our surroundings since then, our stress reaction hasn't altered. Despite its intended use, stress has turned into a chronic illness for a lot of us, negatively impacting our overall health and well-being.

The intricate neuroendocrine system known as the hypothalamic-pituitary-adrenal (HPA) axis is responsible for regulating the stress response. Our hypothalamus releases corticotropin-releasing hormone (CRH) in response to perceived danger, which in turn causes the pituitary gland to produce adrenocorticotropic hormone (ACTH). The production of cortisol and other glucocorticoids by the adrenal glands in reaction to ACTH triggers the stress response. Although the purpose of this complex system is to assist us in responding to dangers, its persistent activation might have unintended effects.

Our bodies go through major physiological changes while we are under stress. Our bodies are primed for action by the release of cortisol, adrenaline, and noradrenaline via hormonal cascades. Increased heart rate, blood pressure, and breathing rate also impact our cardiovascular and respiratory systems, getting our bodies ready for strenuous exercise. Stress also slows down digestion because it diverts blood flow from the stomach to the muscles and other important organs. Although these modifications aid in our reaction to the stressor, persistently triggering the stress response might have negative consequences on our overall health and welfare.

Chronic Stress and Diseases Inflammatory

Persistent stress raises the likelihood of inflammatory disorders and promotes inflammation, both of which may have disastrous implications for our health. Prolonged stress may cause major alterations in immunological function, oxidative stress, and the generation of free radicals, which in turn can contribute to the emergence of several inflammatory disorders linked to stress.

Extended periods of stress lead to the production of pro-inflammatory cytokines, which worsen tissue damage and inflammation. Additionally, stress throws off the immune system's equilibrium, which results in immunological dysregulation and feeds inflammation even more. This leads to a vicious cycle in which stress increases inflammation, which in turn increases stress.

Prolonged stress modifies immune function by increasing the synthesis of pro-inflammatory cytokines and inhibiting the activity of immune cells such as T-cells and natural killer cells. Immune dysregulation results from this, which increases our vulnerability to illnesses and infections. Furthermore, stress encourages immune cell activation, which damages tissue and prolongs inflammation.

Chronic stress also leads to the generation of free radicals and oxidative stress. Stress causes an imbalance between antioxidant defenses and the generation of free radicals, which damages and inflames cells. This may cause harm to different organs and tissues, which might lead to the emergence of inflammatory illnesses.

Numerous inflammatory illnesses, such as cardiovascular disease, gastrointestinal problems like irritable bowel syndrome, autoimmune diseases like lupus and rheumatoid arthritis, and mental health issues like anxiety and depression are all exacerbated by chronic stress. We can reduce the negative impacts of stress and advance general health and well-being by being aware of the connection between chronic stress and inflammation.

Practical Stress-Reduction Methods

Although stress will always exist, there are ways to successfully manage it to greatly enhance general well-being. Numerous methods, each with special advantages and adaptations to suit diverse tastes and lives, may reduce stress. This section explores a variety of stress-reduction techniques, with an emphasis on progressive muscle relaxation, deep breathing exercises, mindfulness and meditation, time management techniques, and nature therapy.

Techniques for Mindfulness and Meditation

Meditation and mindfulness have become quite popular as effective stress-reduction techniques. These techniques promote inner serenity, enhance concentration, and quiet the mind. There are many forms of meditation to suit different requirements and tastes. For example, mindfulness meditation entails paying attention to the here and now while impartially examining thoughts and feelings. It fosters self-awareness and acceptance of one's circumstances. Transcendental meditation, on the other hand, uses silent mantra repetition to help practitioners reach a profound level of awareness and relaxation.

It might be easy to begin a meditation practice. Start by dedicating a short period each day to sit in silence and concentrate on your breathing. Increase the length gradually as you become more at ease. To help newcomers through the procedure, a plethora of applications and internet resources are accessible. Maintaining consistency is essential, and daily meditation practice may develop into a life-changing routine that dramatically lowers stress levels.

Exercises for Deep Breathing

Since breathing exercises directly affect the body's relaxation response, they are also a useful tool for stress management. Deep breathing, also known as diaphragmatic breathing, is taking deep breaths via the nose, letting the belly expand, and then gently releasing the breath through the mouth. This technique may assist in lowering blood pressure, slowing the pulse rate, and fostering calmness.

Box breathing is another widely used method. It entails four counts of inhalation, four counts of holding the breath, four counts of exhalation, and four counts of stopping before repeating. This technique is very helpful for lowering anxiety and enhancing concentration. Regularly putting these strategies into practice will improve your capacity to control stress in daily life.

Gradual Somatic Relaxation

Tensing and then gradually relaxing various bodily muscular groups is known as progressive muscle relaxation or PMR. This technique encourages relaxation and aids in identifying the outward manifestations of stress. To begin practicing PMR, look for a peaceful area to lie down or sit. Starting with your toes, tense and then release the muscles for a brief period. Ascend the body gradually, paying attention to every muscle group.

In addition to relieving stress, PMR may also lessen anxiety symptoms, increase general well-being, and improve the quality of sleep. You may become more conscious of how your body reacts to stress and become more adept at managing it by including PMR in your everyday practice.

Techniques for Time Management

Time management skills are essential for lowering stress since they facilitate juggling several obligations and avoiding overload. Workload management may be effectively achieved with the use of prioritization approaches, such as making to-do lists and grouping jobs according to significance and urgency. Procrastination may be avoided and tension can be decreased by breaking activities down into smaller, more manageable stages.

A well-liked time management strategy is the Pomodoro Technique, which calls for working in concentrated bursts of time—usually 25 minutes—interspersed with brief breaks. This method helps reduce burnout and increase productivity. Digital detox techniques, such as scheduling particular times to check emails and restricting social media usage, may also aid in lowering stress levels and enhancing concentration.

Eco-psychology and Nature Therapy

It has been shown that time spent in nature has many positive effects on both physical and mental health. To lower stress and enhance wellbeing, nature therapy, also known as ecotherapy, entails spending time in the natural world. Engaging in outdoor pursuits like hiking, gardening, or even just strolling through a park may greatly reduce stress and elevate happiness.

Similar advantages may be obtained by city dwellers who incorporate natural components into their everyday lives via outdoor activities, indoor plant maintenance, or trips to nearby parks. Urban nature encounters may provide a much-needed break from the bustle and lessen the negative consequences of city life.

Your general well-being may significantly improve if you include these stress management tactics in your daily routine. Reducing stress may become a more attainable and long-term goal by experimenting with numerous approaches and determining which one suits you the best.

Recognizing When to Seek Professional Help

Although stress is an inherent part of life, it may have detrimental effects on one's physical and emotional well-being when it gets out of control. Maintaining well-being depends on being able to identify when stress is getting out of control and when to get expert assistance. This part will discuss the warning signals of out-of-control stress and the several kinds of professional assistance that may be obtained to help regulate it.

Persistent stress may have a variety of physical and psychological effects. Early symptom recognition may help avoid later, more serious health problems.

Chronic stress may have serious negative bodily implications. One typical symptom is persistent fatigue, which is defined as a persistent sense of exhaustion that does not go away even after receiving enough sleep. There are times when this weariness is so bad that it gets in the way of everyday tasks and productivity. Unknown causes of frequent headaches or migraines are another sign of prolonged stress. These headaches may be migraines, which are more severe and often accompanied by additional symptoms like nausea and sensitivity to light and sound, or tension-type headaches, which are caused by muscular strain.

Tension and soreness in the muscles, especially in the back, shoulders, and neck, are typical physical signs of stress. The body's protracted "fight or flight" reaction causes tension, which over time causes muscles to stay tensed and uncomfortable. Another important physical indicator of ongoing stress is digestive problems. Stress may hurt the gastrointestinal tract, leading to issues including diarrhea, constipation, stomachaches, and irritable bowel syndrome (IBS). These unpleasant sensations are caused by changes in blood flow, secretion, and motility in the stomach caused by stress.

Chronic stress also often results in cardiovascular issues including elevated heart rate, hypertension, or chest discomfort. These symptoms, which raise the risk of heart disease, are brought on by the body's extended exposure to stress chemicals like cortisol and adrenaline. Chronic stress is often accompanied by sleep difficulties, such as trouble getting asleep, staying asleep, or having restless, unrefreshing sleep. Stress is made worse by insomnia or low-quality sleep, which starts a vicious cycle that worsens health.

Frequent infections, colds, and other ailments may result from a compromised immune system brought on by ongoing stress. Stress hormones weaken the immune system, increasing the body's vulnerability to infections and decreasing its capacity to fend against diseases.

Persistent stress has an impact on behavior and mental health as well. An important indicator of persistent anxiety is excessive concern over commonplace events. This anxiety may appear as panic episodes or particular phobias, or it may be widespread. Unmanaged stress may also lead to depression, which is characterized by protracted depressive episodes, despair, or a loss of interest in once-enjoyed activities. Withdrawing from social connections as a result of this emotional state may hurt relationships and quality of life.

You may experience a considerable increase in irritation, rage, or annoyance over trivial matters. Relationships both personally and professionally may be strained by these emotional outbursts, adding to the stress. Chronic stress is typically accompanied by cognitive deficits, such as trouble focusing, making choices, or having memory issues. These cognitive deficiencies result from stress's negative effects on the brain's information-processing and problem-solving abilities.

Another sign may be social distancing and isolation, in which a person isolates themselves from friends and family or avoids social situations. Emotional tiredness and a sense of being overburdened by social commitments often combine to produce this behavior. A major behavioral indicator is increased use of drugs, alcohol, or other substances as a coping technique. While substance misuse reduces stress momentarily, it eventually makes it worse, leading to a vicious cycle of reliance and further health issues.

Weight gain or loss due to significant changes in appetite may be a sign that stress is getting out of control. While some individuals may lose their appetite because of stress-induced sickness or a lack of interest in eating, others may overeat as a consolation.

The first step to getting treatment and taking back control is realizing these symptoms and how they relate to long-term stress. Early intervention may enhance general well-being and stop stress-related health problems from becoming worse.

Available Professional Support Types

When stress gets out of control, expert assistance may provide the coping mechanisms and resources required. There are several solutions to suit a range of requirements and tastes.

Psychotherapy Alternatives

Talk therapy, also referred to as psychotherapy, is a very useful tool for treating chronic stress and its underlying causes. Various therapy modalities may be customized to meet the requirements of each individual:

The goal of **Cognitive Behavioral Therapy (CBT)** is to recognize and alter harmful thinking patterns and actions that lead to stress. It aids in the improvement of coping strategies and problem-solving abilities in people. Goal-oriented and regimented, CBT often includes homework assignments to help clients put new skills into practice in between sessions. It works especially well for sadness and anxiety, two conditions that are often made worse by ongoing stress.

Dialectical Behavior Therapy (DBT): DBT was originally designed to treat borderline personality disorder, but it is also a useful tool for handling stress. It helps people develop resilience by combining mindfulness exercises with cognitive-behavioral therapy to help them control their emotions. To teach skills in four important areas—mindfulness, emotion regulation, distress tolerance, and interpersonal effectiveness—DBT places a strong emphasis on striking a balance between acceptance and change. Those who respond strongly emotionally to stress might benefit from this method.

Acceptance and Commitment Therapy (ACT): ACT promotes accepting one's ideas and emotions as opposed to resisting them. It highlights the dedication to acts in line with individual ideals, encouraging psychological adaptability and stress alleviation. To help people remain present and involved in worthwhile activities even when they are under stress or experiencing unpleasant emotions, ACT uses mindfulness techniques. Chronic stress may be linked to depression, anxiety, and chronic pain, all of which can benefit from this treatment.

Working with an experienced expert who provides individualized ways for coping with stress is known as stress management coaching. Coaches assist clients in identifying stresses and putting into practice practical coping mechanisms by offering direction, responsibility, and support. This strategy may be especially helpful for those who would rather handle their stress in a more planned, goal-oriented manner. Setting clear objectives, creating action plans, and routinely assessing progress are common practices in coaching sessions. In addition, coaches may impart useful skills like stress reduction, time management, and problem-solving methods.

Integrated Medical Methods

Integrative medicine comprehensively approaches stress by fusing unconventional and traditional medical treatments. These methods emphasize the holistic development of the individual, including mental, emotional, and physical health. Among the integrative techniques are:

- Mind-Body Practices: To relieve stress and encourage relaxation, methods like yoga, tai chi, and qigong combine physical exercise with mindfulness and deep breathing. These exercises increase flexibility, promote calmness, and heighten body awareness. Additionally, they have been shown to decrease blood pressure, lessen stress hormones, and enhance mental wellness in general.

Nutritional Counseling: Advice on dietary modifications that promote stress reduction and general health may be obtained from a qualified dietitian or nutritionist. Emotions, energy levels, and the body's capacity to handle stress may all be impacted by proper diet. In addition to specific dietary suggestions to treat any underlying health conditions made worse by stress, nutritional counseling may include advice for a balanced diet high in vitamins, minerals, and antioxidants.

- Acupuncture: To reduce stress and enhance energy flow, tiny needles are inserted into predetermined body locations in this form of traditional Chinese medicine. Acupuncture has been shown to lower stress hormones, elevate mood, and balance the body's energy channels. It may be used alone or in combination with other treatments to improve general health.

- Herbal Medicine: Specific herbs and supplements, including adaptogens, may enhance resilience and assist the body in adjusting to stress. Adaptogens are plant-based compounds that improve the body's capacity to handle stress by controlling physiological functions. Common adaptogens include ginseng, rhodiola, and ashwagandha. Speak with a healthcare professional to ensure safe and efficient usage, particularly when paired with additional therapies.

To improve one's health and well-being, it is proactive to seek expert assistance for stress management. People may choose the best strategy for regaining balance and improving their quality of life by identifying the symptoms of chronic stress and investigating their choices for help. Professional assistance, whether in the form of integrative medicine, coaching, or psychotherapy, offers helpful skills and resources to manage stress better.

By using these expert resources, people may get long-term coping mechanisms to avoid stress in the future in addition to addressing the symptoms of stress that are present right now. This all-encompassing strategy guarantees a more holistic and long-lasting improvement in mental and physical health, which eventually improves quality of life.

Takeaways for Putting Stress Management Strategies Into Practice

Putting stress management strategies into practice calls for a proactive and steady attitude. To start, evaluate yourself to determine which stresses in your life are most prevalent and how they show themselves. Maintaining a diary to monitor your stress levels, physical symptoms, and emotional reactions may assist you in identifying trends and areas that need attention. Make time every day for mindfulness or meditation practice; begin with a short period and work your way up to a longer one. Attend courses or use guided meditation apps to help you develop a regimen.

When you're feeling anxious, try deep breathing techniques like box breathing or diaphragmatic breathing. To help you manage stress proactively, include these exercises in your everyday routine, for example, before bed or throughout your morning routine. Set aside time every day to do Progressive Muscle Relaxation (PMR) exercises. Locate a peaceful, comfortable area where you can concentrate on tensing and releasing your muscle groups. To guarantee proper execution, use step-by-step instructions or audio tutorials.

Use time management strategies to lessen the stress brought on by excessive workloads. Use techniques such as the Eisenhower Matrix to prioritize your duties, the Pomodoro Technique to divide your work into concentrated periods, and frequent breaks to avoid burnout. Establishing limits for technology usage, such as a screen time restriction or designated tech-free areas inside your house, might help you consider going through a digital detox. Establish the routine of spending time in nature. Make nature therapy a part of your weekly routine, whether it's taking a stroll in the park, going on a hike, or just relaxing in your garden. Urbanites may visit parks and botanical gardens, or they can bring nature home with plants and décor that draw inspiration from it.

Do not be afraid to get expert assistance if you see symptoms of chronic stress. Speak with a therapist about your possibilities for psychotherapy, or work with a stress management coach to create specialized plans. Integrative medicine techniques may be used in conjunction with conventional therapy to provide a comprehensive approach to stress management. Make connections with friends, family, or support groups to create a solid support network. You may get both practical stress management solutions and emotional comfort by talking about your experiences and asking others for help.

You may start incorporating stress-reduction strategies into your everyday life and develop a more resilient and well-rounded approach to managing stress by implementing these action steps. You will develop resilience and enhance your general well-being by using these tactics daily, so consistency and dedication are essential. Stress management is a continuous process, therefore it's critical to periodically assess your methods and modify them to meet your changing requirements.

3. NUTRITION

Feeding Your Microbiome

Keeping the gut healthy is critical for general health since the gut is involved in immune system function, nutrition absorption, and digestion. Dietary assistance is possible for a healthy gut microbiome, which is made up of billions of beneficial bacteria. Fermented foods and foods high in prebiotics are two important dietary elements that support a healthy gut.

Foods High in Prebiotics

Prebiotics are indigestible fibers that feed the good bacteria in the stomach. Prebiotics support the growth of these bacteria, which is necessary for the proper balance of gut flora and overall digestive health. Foods high in prebiotics include:

Onions and Garlic: A kind of prebiotic fiber called inulin may be found in abundance in these veggies. Onions and garlic not only provide food taste, but they also encourage the formation of good intestinal flora. To preserve their prebiotic properties, eat them raw or very gently cooked.

Jerusalem artichokes and asparagus: These two veggies are high in prebiotic fibers, including inulin. While Jerusalem artichokes, also referred to as sunchokes, are good roasted or added to soups, asparagus is best served grilled, steamed, or mixed into salads.

Cucumbers: Bananas are an excellent source of resistant starch, which is a kind of prebiotic fiber, especially when they are somewhat green. Eating bananas may assist enhance intestinal health by encouraging the development of good bacteria.

Barley and Oats: Prebiotic soluble fiber known as beta-glucan is found in whole grains such as barley and oats. Including these grains in your diet helps promote a balanced microbiota in your stomach. Use barley as a side dish or in soups, and enjoy oats as oatmeal or in smoothies.

Apples: Pectin is a soluble fiber that functions as a prebiotic and may be found in apples. By encouraging the development of good bacteria, eating apples with their skin on may enhance intestinal health.

Onion: Leeks are high in inulin, much like onions and garlic. They give a subtle onion flavor and prebiotic benefits to a variety of foods, and they may be utilized in soups, stews, or other culinary applications.

You may encourage the development and activity of good gut bacteria by including these foods high in prebiotics in your diet. This can help to increase immunity, aid with digestion, and support general health.

Fermented Foods

Probiotics, or live beneficial bacteria, are abundant in fermented foods and help maintain a healthy gut microbiota. Eating fermented foods may improve immunity and improve digestive health by repopulating and diversifying the gut flora. Popular foods that are fermented include:

Yogurt: One of the most popular probiotic foods is yogurt. Yogurt is a fermented milk product that has a high concentration of Lactobacillus and Bifidobacterium, two kinds of helpful bacteria. To avoid additional sugars, choose plain, unsweetened yogurt and search for products that indicate live, active cultures on the label.

Kefir: Kefir is a fermented milk beverage with a wide variety of probiotics, much like yogurt. Its thinner consistency and acidic taste make it ideal for both standalone refreshing drinks and smoothies.

Crue: Finely shredded cabbage is fermented with lactic acid bacteria to make sauerkraut. This crunchy, tart condiment is full of probiotics and tastes great as a side dish or added to salads and sandwiches.

Kimchi: Kimchi, a spicy fermented vegetable dish prepared usually with cabbage, radishes, and a variety of spices, is a mainstay of Korean cuisine. Rich in Lactobacillus bacteria, kimchi may be used as a flavoring for a variety of foods or consumed on its own.

Kombucha: Kombucha is a tea beverage that undergoes fermentation with the addition of a symbiotic culture of yeast and bacteria (SCOBY) to sweetened tea. Enjoy this pleasant probiotic-rich fizzy drink as a healthy substitute for sugar-filled drinks.

Miso: A prominent ingredient in Japanese cuisine is miso, a fermented soybean paste. It may be used to produce marinades, sauces, and miso soup. It is also rich in beneficial microorganisms. Consuming miso may improve intestinal health and give food a distinct umami taste.

Tempeh: Tempeh is a hard, nutty-flavored food made from fermented soybeans. It is a fantastic source of plant-based protein and works well in a variety of recipes, including salads, sandwiches, and stir-fries. Soybeans' probiotic content is increased and their nutrients are more easily absorbed during the fermentation process.

Crunchy potatoes: Pickles that are naturally fermented and produced without vinegar are a great way to get probiotics. To find pickles with beneficial bacteria, look for those that are labeled as organically fermented or brined. Savor them as a snack or include them in salads and sandwiches.

By including fermented foods in your diet, you may promote a varied and healthy microbiome in your stomach by introducing beneficial bacteria. This may thus strengthen the immune system, facilitate better digestion, and promote general health. Fermented foods and prebiotic-rich meals work together to provide a synergistic impact that supports gut health and well-being at its best.

Fiber's Function in Fostering Beneficial Bacteria

To maintain a healthy digestive system and general well-being, fiber is vital for fostering good microorganisms in the stomach. You may choose a diet that supports healthy gut flora by being aware of the various forms of fiber and how they affect gut health.

Soluble and insoluble fiber are the two main forms of fiber and each has unique advantages for gut health.

Soluble Fiber turns into a gel-like material in the digestive track when it dissolves in water. This kind of fiber may be found in foods including citrus fruits, apples, beans, and oats. In the gut, soluble fiber is very helpful for fostering good bacteria. The gut bacteria ferment it as it moves through the digestive system, resulting in the production of short-chain fatty acids (SCFAs) such as butyrate, acetate, and propionate. These SCFAs support a strong gut barrier, aid in the regulation of inflammation, and provide the cells lining the gut with a source of energy. Furthermore, by delaying the absorption of glucose, soluble fiber lowers blood sugar levels, which is advantageous for maintaining metabolic health and controlling weight.

Contrarily, Insoluble Fiber does not dissolve in water and gives the stool more volume, which helps to encourage regular bowel movements and ward against constipation. Insoluble fiber, which may be found in foods like whole grains, nuts, seeds, and vegetables, aids in maintaining digestive health by accelerating the passage of food through the digestive system and boosting the volume of stool. Even while insoluble fiber does not ferment as quickly as soluble fiber, it still contributes to gut motility and health, which helps to create an environment that is conducive for beneficial bacteria.

For a diet that promotes gut health and is well-rounded, both forms of fiber are essential. Maintaining an equilibrium between soluble and insoluble fiber guarantees that you get the distinct benefits of each kind, therefore fostering a vibrant and varied gut microbiota.

Suggested Daily Consumption of Fiber

The amount of fiber that should be consumed each day varies based on age, gender, and personal health requirements. Dietary standards recommend that individuals strive to ingest around 25 grams of fiber per day for women and 38 grams for men to promote overall health. Based on the average quantity required to sustain healthy gut flora, encourage digestive health, and lower the risk of chronic illnesses, these recommendations have been made.

Make an effort to include a range of foods high in fiber in your diet to reach these fiber consumption targets. Consuming an abundance of fruits, vegetables, whole grains, legumes, nuts, and seeds is part of this. For example, you may get a good amount of your daily fiber intake by beginning your day with a bowl of oatmeal topped with a handful of nuts and fresh fruit. Other ways to increase your intake of fiber include adding beans or lentils to salads and soups, selecting whole-grain goods over refined grains, and having fresh fruits or vegetables as a snack.

Drink plenty of water and gradually increase your intake of fiber to assist your digestive system adapt and avoiding discomforts like gas and bloating. Making abrupt changes to your fiber intake might cause digestive problems, so it's important to go slowly so your stomach can acclimate.

It is important to have a range of dietary sources of fiber to get the benefits of both soluble and insoluble fiber. This method supports proper digestion, fosters the growth of beneficial bacteria, and advances gut health in general. Following the suggested daily fiber intake and including foods high in fiber in your diet can help you maintain a healthy, balanced gut microbiota that benefits your general health.

Curcumin with Anti-Inflammatory Herbs

The Top 10 Spices to Reduce Inflammation

Including spices that are anti-inflammatory in your diet may make a big difference in lowering inflammation and improving general health. Numerous of these spices include active ingredients that have a range of health advantages, from strengthening immune system function to lowering oxidative stress. Ten of the best anti-inflammatory spices, their advantages, and their active ingredients are listed below:

1. Turmeric

Due mainly to its active ingredient, curcumin, turmeric is well-known for both its vivid yellow color and its anti-inflammatory qualities. It has been shown that curcumin inhibits inflammatory pathways and lowers the body's concentration of inflammatory markers. Additionally, it has antioxidant qualities that aid in reducing oxidative stress and neutralizing free radicals. In addition to these health benefits, turmeric may improve the taste of smoothies, soups, and curries.

2. Ginger

Gingerol, one of the bioactive chemicals in ginger, is what gives it its anti-inflammatory properties. It has been discovered that gingerol reduces inflammation and discomfort by inhibiting the production of pro-inflammatory cytokines and enzymes. In addition to providing digestive health benefits, ginger may enhance the taste of teas, stir-fries, and marinades.

3. Onion

Garlic's sulfur-containing chemicals, such as allicin, are primarily responsible for its anti-inflammatory qualities. Through the modulation of many inflammatory pathways, allicin has been shown to decrease inflammation and enhance immunological function. From sautés to sauces, garlic is a versatile ingredient that works well in a variety of recipes.

4. Cinnamon

An important ingredient in cinnamon that adds to its anti-inflammatory and antioxidant qualities is cinnamaldehyde. Cinnamaldehyde has been shown to enhance blood sugar management and decrease inflammation by blocking inflammatory cytokines. For a toasty, sweet taste, add cinnamon to smoothies, baked goods, and cereal.

5. Cayenne pepper

Capsaicin, a substance found in cayenne pepper, has anti-inflammatory and analgesic properties. Capsaicin increases the body's capacity to tolerate pain by decreasing the synthesis of chemicals that cause inflammation. Cayenne pepper is a prominent component in spicy sauces and spice mixes, and it may be used to impart heat to food.

6. Rosemary

Rosmarinic acid, a substance with potent anti-inflammatory and antioxidant qualities, is abundant in rosemary. Rosmarinic acid enhances general immunological health by assisting in the inhibition of pro-inflammatory enzyme activity. Fresh or dried rosemary adds taste and health benefits to meats, veggies, and baked items.

7. Thyme

Thymol and carvacrol are two of the active ingredients in thyme that contribute to its antibacterial and anti-inflammatory qualities. It has been shown that thymol lowers inflammation and promotes respiratory health. One of the most adaptable herbs, thyme works well in marinades, stews, and soups.

8. Oregano

Carvacrol and rosmarinic acid, in particular, are abundant anti-inflammatory and antioxidant substances found in oregano. These substances aid in lowering the body's oxidative stress and inflammation. In addition to its health advantages, oregano may lend a powerful taste to Mediterranean recipes, sauces, and dressings.

9. Cloves

Eugenol, a substance with strong analgesic and anti-inflammatory qualities, is found in cloves. Cloves are a great complement to anti-inflammatory diets because they contain eugenol, which reduces inflammation and relieves pain. Cloves may be used for savory recipes, baked items, and spice mixes.

10. Black Pepper

Piperine, an active ingredient in black pepper, improves the absorption of other health-promoting substances like turmeric and curcumin. In addition to its anti-inflammatory qualities, piperine promotes intestinal health. A popular ingredient for everything from soups to meat meals is black pepper.

How to Incorporate Anti-Inflammatory Seasonings into Your Diet

Including spices that reduce inflammation in your diet may improve taste and have health advantages. You can optimize the health advantages of these spices by knowing the best ways to prepare them and how to take supplements. Here's how to successfully include them in your meals:

Cooking Methods to Increase Benefits

1. Use Fresh and Dried Herbs and Spices: To retain their volatile oils and active compounds, fresh herbs such as basil, thyme, and rosemary may be added to recipes at the end of cooking. To let the taste of the dried herbs and spices, such as cloves, cinnamon, and turmeric, seep into the food, add them at the start of cooking.

2. Combine with Healthy Fats: Since many anti-inflammatory substances are fat-soluble, eating them with healthy fats improves their absorption. For example, curcumin, the active ingredient in turmeric, works best when combined with lipids like coconut or olive oil. Consider adding a small quantity of healthy fat to recipes that call for turmeric or other fat-soluble spices to improve absorption.

3. Avoid Overheating: Certain herbs and spices lose their power when heated excessively. For example, cooking garlic for an extended period at a high temperature might cause it to lose some of its healthful properties. To preserve the health advantages of garlic, add it at the end of cooking or use it raw in sauces and dressings.

4. Use in a range of recipes: To routinely get the advantages of these spices, include them in a range of recipes. Use garlic and ginger in stir-fries and marinades, add turmeric to soups and stews, and sprinkle cinnamon over porridge or yogurt. You may figure out the best methods to include these flavors into your diet by experimenting with various foods.

5. Prepare Teas and Infusions: Use spices, ginger, and turmeric to make teas or infusions that reduce inflammation. All you need to do is soak these spices in hot water to create a calming and beneficial drink. You may improve the taste and health benefits by adding a little honey or a squeeze of lemon.

6. Blend into Smoothies: For an additional health boost, smoothies may benefit from the addition of certain anti-inflammatory spices. To your favorite smoothie recipe, add a bit of turmeric, a couple of slices of fresh ginger, or a sprinkle of cinnamon. This is a simple way to add these ingredients to your everyday meals.

Doses and Forms of Supplements

Although adding spices to your food is good for you, supplements may provide concentrated forms of these compounds—particularly if you need larger quantities for medical reasons. Here's how to make good use of supplements:

1. Turmeric/Curcumin Supplements: Supplements containing turmeric come in a range of formats, such as powders, pills, and capsules. To improve absorption, look for pills that include piperine, or black pepper extract, with curcumin. Curcumin doses typically vary from 500 to 2000 mg daily. Before raising the dosage, always start with a smaller one and speak with your doctor, particularly if you take other drugs or have health issues.

2. Ginger Supplements: Tablets and pills are the most prevalent forms of ginger supplements. The usual range of standard doses is 500–1000 mg daily. You may also get ginger in liquid extract form to use in tea or water. To ascertain the ideal dose for your requirements, speak with a healthcare professional.

3. Garlic Supplements: Garlic supplements come in a variety of forms, such as oil, pills, and odorless capsules. The usual doses of garlic extract are 600–1200 mg daily. For dependable results, look for products with standardized allicin content.

4. Cinnamon Supplements: Standard doses for cinnamon supplements typically range from 500 to 1000 mg daily. Supplements are available in pill form. Make sure you use supplements made with Ceylon cinnamon instead of Cassia cinnamon since the latter might have greater concentrations of coumarin, which can be dangerous in excess.

5. Capsaicin Supplements: Available in topical or pill forms, capsaicin is a compound present in cayenne pepper. Doses for oral supplements typically fall between 30 and 120 mg daily. Topical lotions containing capsaicin are another option for treating localized pain.

6. Oregano, Thyme, and Rosemary Supplements: These herbs are often offered as extracts or capsules. Doses might vary, therefore for individualized advice, refer to the manufacturer's instructions and speak with a healthcare professional.

It's important to use supplements according to suggested quantities and see a doctor, particularly if you have underlying medical concerns or are on other drugs. By including these anti-inflammatory ingredients in your meals via cooking and supplements, you may promote general health and efficiently control inflammation.

How to Recognize Inflammatory Foods

An important factor in controlling inflammation in the body is diet. Some dietary ingredients may function as catalysts, encouraging inflammatory processes that might result in long-term health problems. Knowing these typical food triggers can empower you to make well-informed decisions that will lower inflammation and promote general health.

Refined Sugars and Corn Syrup with High Fructose

High-fructose corn syrup (HFCS) and refined sugars are common ingredients in a lot of processed meals and sugary drinks. These compounds may aggravate inflammation in several ways. Refined sweets raise blood glucose levels when ingested in excess, which increases oxidative stress and the production of inflammatory cytokines. Because of its high fructose content, which may worsen insulin resistance and encourage chronic inflammation, high-fructose corn syrup—which is often found in sodas and processed snacks—is especially worrisome. Cutting less on drinks, sugar-filled snacks, and sugary meals will help reduce inflammation and enhance metabolic health.

Hydrogenated and Trans Fats

Fast food, baked products, and processed and fried foods like margarine are common sources of trans fats and hydrogenated oils. These fats are produced by an industrial method that solidifies and stabilizes liquid vegetable oils by adding hydrogen. Trans fats are known to cause an imbalance that fuels inflammation and advances cardiovascular disease by raising levels of low-density lipoprotein (LDL) cholesterol and lowering levels of high-density lipoprotein (HDL) cholesterol. Selecting heart-healthy fats, like those in nuts, avocados, and olive oil, may help lower inflammation and promote cardiac health.

Overabundance of Omega-6 Fatty Acids

Essential fats and omega-6 fatty acids are involved in the operation of cell membranes and general health. However, they might cause inflammation if taken in excess in comparison to omega-3 fatty acids. Vegetable oils, including sunflower, soybean, and maize oils, are rich sources of omega-6 fatty acids and are often used in processed meals. An imbalance between omega-3 and omega-6 fatty acids may cause pro-inflammatory molecules to be produced. Reduce your consumption of processed oils high in omega-6 fatty acids and increase your consumption of omega-3-rich foods like walnuts, flaxseeds, and fatty fish to achieve a balanced omega-6 to omega-3 ratio.

Refined Sugars and Carbs

Refined carbs are derived from highly processed grains that have had their fiber and nutrients removed. Examples of these foods include white bread, pastries, and many morning cereals. These meals raise blood sugar levels quickly, which exacerbates oxidative stress and inflammation. Additionally, refined carbs may lead to weight gain, which aggravates inflammatory diseases. Choosing whole grains offers more nutrients and fiber, which helps to lower inflammation and regulate blood sugar levels. Examples of whole grains include brown rice, quinoa, and whole-wheat products.

Through the identification and mitigation of these prevalent food triggers, you may make dietary decisions that facilitate your body's capacity to regulate inflammation. A balanced diet high in fiber, healthy fats, and whole foods may help sustain a normal inflammatory response and enhance general health.

How to Gradually Cut Out Inflammatory Foods

Reducing inflammation and enhancing general health may both be achieved by cutting out inflammatory items from your diet. On the other hand, you may adapt more readily and sustain long-term success if you make these adjustments gradually. Here's a detailed tutorial on how to progressively cut out inflammatory foods, along with some helpful hints for properly reading food labels.

A Comprehensive Removal Procedure

- Identify Foods That Cause Inflammation: Make a list of the typical items that cause inflammation and that you wish to avoid, such as refined sugars, trans fats, high-fructose corn syrup, and processed carbs. Keeping a food journal for a week might be useful to see trends and identify certain foods you eat a lot of.
- Set Clear Goals: Establish reasonable objectives for the removal procedure. For instance, you may choose to cut out a certain kind of inflammatory food once a week or concentrate on cutting down by a specific percentage. Establishing clear, attainable objectives can assist you in staying on course and making little changes over time.
- Initiate Minor Adjustments: Start by modifying your diet in tiny, doable steps. If you're trying to cut out refined sugars, for example, start by giving up sugary beverages and switching to herbal teas or water. Reduce the amount of sugary snacks and desserts you consume gradually over time.
- Substitute with Healthier Alternatives: Choose healthier alternatives to foods that cause inflammation. For example, use whole grains like brown rice or quinoa in place of processed carbs. Instead of trans fats and hydrogenated oils, use healthy fats like avocado or olive oil. Selecting whole, unprocessed meals may support your health objectives while helping you satiate urges.

- Monitor Your Progress: Keep tabs on your development and record any improvements in your emotional state. Pay attention to any changes in your general health, digestion, or energy levels. Based on your observations and the input from your body, modify your strategy as necessary.
- Seek Support and Stay Informed: You may want to think about getting in touch with a dietitian or nutritionist who can guide you through the elimination process and provide individualized recommendations. Continue your education by reading about health and nutrition, since this may inspire you and provide you with fresh suggestions for sticking to a well-balanced, anti-inflammatory diet.
- Be Patient and Persistent: Keep in mind that giving up foods that cause inflammation takes time. Give yourself time and patience so that your habits and taste senses can change. Persistence is essential, and over time, even little adjustments may have a big positive impact on your health.

Effectively Reading Food Labels

1. Verify the list of ingredients Check the ingredients list for items that are known to cause inflammation, such as hydrogenated oils, processed sugars, and high-fructose corn syrup. The order of ingredients is based on their weight, therefore the more an ingredient is listed higher, the more of it there is in the final product.

2. Identify Added Sugars : Know that added sugars go by several names, including maltose, glucose, sucrose, and dextrose. Additionally, look for words like "nectar" or "syrup," which suggest the addition of sugar. Try to choose goods that have little or no added sugar.

3. Look for Healthy Fats: Make sure the product is free of hydrogenated or trans fats. The quantity of trans fats per serving will be given on the nutrition information label, and hydrogenated oils can be included in the ingredients list. Choose goods like avocado or olive oil that are high in healthful fats.

4. Check the Fiber Level: Select goods with more fiber as it supports intestinal health and helps to normalize blood sugar levels. Seek whole grains and those with the label "high in fiber."

5. Review Serving Sizes: Take note of the serving sizes that are shown on the label with the nutrition statistics. Sometimes items with tiny serving sizes seem healthier, but if they include substances that cause inflammation, larger portion amounts taken in real life might exacerbate inflammation.

6. Understand Nutrition Claims: Pay close attention to any health claims made on the package, such as "low-fat" or "sugar-free." These statements do not imply that the product is devoid of inflammatory components. To get a clear picture of what you're eating, always review the nutrition information and the whole ingredient list.

You may progressively cut out inflammatory items from your diet and replace them with healthier options by following these guidelines and making good use of food labels. This procedure may help lower inflammation, enhance general health, and establish nutritional habits that will last a lifetime and promote your well-being.

Exploring Anti-Inflammatory Diets

Eating regimens that target inflammation may provide several methods for lowering inflammation and promoting general health. Various strategies have different advantages and are supported to differing degrees by scientific data. This is a summary of a few well-known anti-inflammatory diets, contrasting their methods and looking at the data from science to back them up.

Mediterranean Diet

The advantages of the Mediterranean diet in reducing inflammation are well known. It limits red meat and processed foods and emphasizes whole, unprocessed foods such as fish, poultry, lean meat, fruits, vegetables, whole grains, nuts, and seeds. This diet contains omega-3 fatty acids from fish, which are believed to have anti-inflammatory qualities, as well as healthy fats from nuts and olive oil that help lower inflammation. The efficacy of the Mediterranean diet in decreasing inflammatory markers and lowering the risk of chronic illnesses like diabetes and heart disease is supported by scientific research.

DASH Diet

Created to treat high blood pressure, the Dietary Approaches to Stop Hypertension (DASH) diet also has anti-inflammatory properties. It involves consuming less added sweets, red meat, saturated fats, and whole grains in addition to a high consumption of fruits, vegetables, lean meats, and low-fat dairy. The emphasis on nutrient-rich meals and minimal salt consumption in this diet helps control blood pressure and reduce inflammation. Studies indicate that the DASH diet is a useful tool for lowering blood pressure and reducing inflammation, both of which improve cardiovascular health in general.

Paleo Diet

This diet emphasizes consuming no grains, legumes, dairy products, or processed foods, and instead focuses on eating as our pre-agricultural ancestors did by emphasizing lean meats, fish, fruits, vegetables, nuts, and seeds. Reduced inflammation is the goal of the Paleo diet, which excludes refined and processed foods. It highlights foods high in omega-3, such as nuts and seafood. The data on the Paleo diet's potential to lower inflammation and enhance metabolic health is conflicting, and eliminating whole food categories may result in nutrient shortages.

Whole30 Diet

The Whole30 diet is a thirty-day plan aimed at removing foods that may cause inflammation and other health problems. It emphasizes entire, unprocessed foods—such as nuts, fruits, vegetables, meats, and seafood—while avoiding grains, legumes, dairy, sugar, and alcohol. This brief period of elimination aids in the identification of certain dietary sensitivities and how they affect inflammation. Nevertheless, there is no long-term data to support the Whole30 regimen, and not everyone may be able to adhere to its tight guidelines.

The anti-inflammatory diet is a more adaptable and individualized strategy that emphasizes eating foods like fruits, vegetables, whole grains, nuts, seeds, and lean meats that are proven to lower inflammation. Its main goal is to consume less processed meals, refined carbohydrates, and harmful fats. This diet offers a well-rounded strategy for lowering inflammation by including components of both the DASH and Mediterranean diets. There is scientific proof that an anti-inflammatory diet may effectively lower inflammation and enhance general health.

Selecting the appropriate eating plan is based on dietary requirements, personal preferences, and health objectives. Combining components of these diets may promote long-term health and help lower inflammation.

The Autoimmune Protocol (AIP)

By identifying and eliminating items that may cause immune reactions, the Autoimmune Protocol (AIP) diet is a customized elimination diet intended to treat autoimmune disorders and decrease inflammation. The AIP emphasizes nutrient-dense, anti-inflammatory foods while avoiding those that can exacerbate immune system dysfunction, to repair the gut and lower systemic inflammation.

Foods to Avoid: AIP diets exclude several items that are believed to trigger the immune system or cause inflammation. These consist of nightshade vegetables (tomatoes, peppers, eggplants, and potatoes), cereals, legumes, dairy products, refined sugars, and processed meals. Furthermore, chemicals and seed oils that might irritate or worsen inflammation in the gut lining are prohibited from the diet.

Foods to Include: The diet places a strong emphasis on nutrient-dense foods that lower inflammation and promote intestinal health. These consist of a range of veggies (apart from nightshades), fruits, seafood, organ meats, premium meats, and healthy fats like olive and coconut oils. It's also advised to include fermented foods, since these may help repair the stomach.

The AIP Phases

Elimination Phase: The first step is eliminating anything that can cause inflammation or allergies from the diet. This phase, which usually lasts 30 to 60 days, is all about eating only foods that are compatible with the AIP. Giving the gut and immune systems time to recover while lowering general inflammation is the aim. People regularly monitor their symptoms throughout this period, and they can see improvements in their overall health and well-being.

Reintroduction Phase: Following the elimination phase, people progressively reintroduce the items they had removed one at a time to see which ones could cause negative responses. Over several days, each meal is gradually reintroduced back in while any symptom changes are closely monitored. Through this procedure, particular food sensitivities may be identified and a long-term dietary plan that reduces inflammatory reactions can be customized.

Maintenance Phase: Following the identification of food sensitivities, people go onto a maintenance phase in which they concentrate on eating a balanced diet that includes a greater range of foods while avoiding recognized triggers. The goal of this phase is to sustain the gains made during the elimination phase and provide long-term management of autoimmune symptoms.

People may try to reduce inflammation, repair the gut, and better manage autoimmune disorders by adhering to the tenets and stages of the AIP diet. Nutrient-dense foods are prioritized in the AIP method, which offers a systematic framework for detecting and managing dietary triggers to improve general health.

Individuals Who Can Gain from the Autoimmune Protocol (AIP) Method

People with autoimmune diseases are the main target audience for the Autoimmune Protocol (AIP) diet. People who suffer from conditions including lupus, celiac disease, rheumatoid arthritis, and Hashimoto's thyroiditis may find it very helpful. AIP seeks to lessen symptoms related to these illnesses by concentrating on lowering inflammation and repairing the gut. The diet's focus on nutrient-dense, anti-inflammatory foods aids in addressing immune system dysfunction at its root and improves the management of flare-ups. According to research and anecdotal data, many autoimmune patients find that adhering to the AIP diet reduces their symptoms and improves their quality of life.

Even though there are a lot of advantages to the AIP diet, there are certain hazards to be aware of. The diet's restriction, which may result in nutritional deficits if not well handled, is one of the main causes of worry. For instance, cutting out whole food categories like dairy and grains may lead to a decrease in the consumption of vital minerals like fiber, calcium, and B vitamins. To prevent deficits, it is essential to keep a diverse and well-balanced diet within the AIP framework.

The possibility of heightened sensitivity or intolerance to food during the reintroduction stage is another factor to take into account. People may encounter new symptoms or responses as they progressively reintroduce items they had removed, which may be difficult to control. Working with a nutritionist or healthcare professional and maintaining thorough documentation can make this process easier to handle.

Furthermore, adhering to the AIP diet's rigorous elimination phase, which calls for considerable adjustments to eating patterns and meal preparation, may be difficult. This stage may also be difficult socially since it calls for avoiding a lot of familiar meals and substances. Managing these obstacles may benefit from the assistance of support groups and medical specialists.

Finally, even though the AIP diet may help a lot of people, it might not be the best option for everyone. Before beginning the diet, those with certain medical issues or those taking particular drugs should speak with their healthcare professional. The diet may be made to be both safe and successful by collaborating with a healthcare provider and tailoring the strategy to each person's unique health requirements.

Benefits of a Mediterranean Diet

Many people recognize the health advantages of the Mediterranean diet, especially its ability to reduce inflammation. The following are some essential elements and study results on its beneficial effects on inflammation and general health:

Plant-Based Foods Are Stressed Out: The Mediterranean diet's emphasis on plant-based meals is one of its most characteristic features. A diet rich in fruits, vegetables, whole grains, legumes, nuts, and seeds is part of this. These foods are high in fiber, antioxidants, vitamins, and minerals—all of which help to lower inflammation. A spectrum of phytonutrients that fight oxidative stress and inflammation may be found in fruits like berries, oranges, and apples, as well as vegetables like leafy greens, tomatoes, and peppers.

Healthy Fats and Lean Proteins: Olive oil, a mainstay of Mediterranean cooking, is one of the best sources of healthy fats in the Mediterranean diet. Rich in monounsaturated fats, olive oil also includes antioxidants such as oleocanthal, which functions as an ibuprofen-like anti-inflammatory. The diet also contains modest quantities of lean proteins, mostly from chicken and fish. Fish that are high in fat, including salmon, mackerel, and sardines, are great providers of omega-3 fatty acids, which have potent anti-inflammatory properties. Nuts and seeds are another source of protein and good fats in the diet.

The Mediterranean diet has been shown in several studies to be very effective in lowering the risk of cardiovascular illnesses, which are often brought on by chronic inflammation. Studies show that this diet helps reduce inflammatory indicators including interleukin-6 (IL-6) and C-reactive protein (CRP). A substantial reduction in the risk of severe cardiovascular events, such as heart attack, stroke, and cardiovascular mortality, was seen in those who followed a Mediterranean diet supplemented with extra-virgin olive oil or nuts, according to the PREDIMED trial, seminal research. The diet's focus on foods high in fiber, antioxidants, and healthy fats improves blood pressure, lipid profiles, and heart health in general.

The Mediterranean diet has anti-inflammatory benefits that also benefit mental health. It is thought that neurodegenerative illnesses like Alzheimer's and other types of dementia are influenced by inflammation in their early stages. According to research, following a Mediterranean diet is linked to a decreased risk of Alzheimer's disease and a slower pace of cognitive decline. The abundance of anti-inflammatory and antioxidant-rich foods in the diet helps shield brain tissue from oxidative stress and inflammation, which may otherwise cause cognitive decline. Additionally, by lowering neuroinflammation and encouraging the preservation of neuronal function, omega-3 fatty acids, which are present in fatty fish, improve brain health.

In addition to its effects on cardiovascular and cognitive health, studies have connected the Mediterranean diet to improved gut health, better control of type 2 diabetes, and a decreased risk of some malignancies. The anti-inflammatory characteristics of the diet aid in reducing the chronic inflammation that often accompanies these ailments. For instance, eating a diet rich in fiber helps to maintain a healthy gut flora, which is essential for controlling inflammation throughout the body. Additionally, the low glycemic index of the diet contributes to stable blood sugar levels and lowers insulin resistance-related inflammation.

Plant-Based Eating

Plant nutrients, also known as phytonutrients, are substances that have potent anti-inflammatory properties and are present in fruits, vegetables, grains, beans, nuts, and seeds. These include the antioxidants flavonoids, carotenoids, and polyphenols, which help the body fight oxidative stress and inflammation. Berries, apples, and onions are rich sources of flavonoids, which have anti-inflammatory and anti-inflammatory properties. Carotenoids, which include lycopene in tomatoes and beta-carotene in carrots, are antioxidants that reduce inflammation. It has been shown that polyphenols, which are found in large amounts in foods like dark chocolate, green tea, and grapes, decrease inflammation by preventing the synthesis of inflammatory chemicals. You may strengthen your body's defenses against inflammation and reduce your chance of developing chronic illnesses by eating a range of plant foods high in these phytonutrients.

Making the switch to plant-based proteins may dramatically lower inflammation. Plant-based proteins are often low in saturated fat and rich in fiber and antioxidants, in contrast to animal proteins, which might exacerbate inflammation because of their high saturated fat concentration. Legumes are high in protein, fiber, and important minerals. Examples of legumes include beans, lentils, and chickpeas. Nuts and seeds, such as flaxseeds, chia seeds, walnuts, and almonds, provide heart-healthy lipids in addition to protein. Because they are high in protein and other minerals, whole grains like buckwheat, farro, and quinoa are perfect for a plant-based diet. These protein sources may improve long-term health outcomes by boosting the maintenance of muscle mass, supporting metabolic health, and reducing general inflammation.

Changing to a Plant-Based Diet

Strategy for Meal Planning: Meal planning is essential to making the switch to a plant-based diet effective. Aim for a couple of meatless days each week and begin by progressively adding more plant-based meals to your diet. Make sure to center your meals on healthy grains, legumes, nuts, seeds, and veggies. Try bulk cooking and prepping meals to save time and make sure you have wholesome alternatives accessible. Try experimenting with different dishes to maintain an interesting and well-balanced diet. For instance, you might make a huge pot of stewed vegetables, a large salad made of quinoa, or a tray of roasted veggies that you could eat for many meals over the week. Breakfast alternatives may include a smoothie prepared with bananas, almond milk, and leafy greens, or overnight oats topped with fresh berries and almonds. Think of robust salads, grain bowls, stir-fried vegetables, and meals made with legumes, such as chickpea curry or lentil soup, for lunch and supper. Having a well-stocked pantry with essentials like whole grains, beans, lentils, nuts, and seeds can help you stay on track with your plant-based eating objectives and make meal preparation easier.

Plant-Based Substitutes for Frequently Used Animal Products: One of the difficulties in switching to a plant-based diet is finding appropriate animal product substitutes. Thankfully, there are many plant-based substitutes for meat, dairy, and eggs that work just as well. Tofu, tempeh, seitan, or plant-based meat alternatives derived from soy or pea protein are good options for protein. Almond milk, soy milk, oat milk, and coconut milk are dairy substitutes that work similarly to cow's milk in baking and cooking. In addition to having a cheesy taste, nutritional yeast is a fantastic cheese alternative and a strong source of B vitamins. For eggs, look into recipes for tofu scrambles as a savory breakfast alternative. You can also try using flaxseeds or chia seeds combined with water as a binding agent in baking. You may cut less on animal products while still maintaining a balanced diet by including these plant-based substitutes.

Making the switch to a plant-based diet is good for the environment as well as your health. Plant-based protein sources and an emphasis on phytonutrient-rich plant foods will help you decrease inflammation and enhance your general health. Transitioning to plant-based alternatives to popular animal products and meal planning may help make the process easier and more pleasurable. Adopting a plant-based diet is a step in the right direction for a more sustainable planet and a better way of living.

Getting Rid of Gluten

The protein gluten is present in wheat, barley, and rye. Some individuals may get serious health problems as a result of eating gluten. Gluten consumption causes damage to the small intestine in those with celiac disease, an autoimmune condition. When people with celiac disease consume gluten, their small intestine's lining is attacked by their immune system, which results in inflammation and impairs the absorption of vital nutrients. Anemia, weariness, joint pain, and digestive problems are some of the symptoms associated with celiac disease.

Conversely, non-celiac gluten sensitivity (NCGS) is a condition in which people have symptoms including headaches, bloating, and stomach discomfort, but without the immunological reaction or intestinal damage associated with celiac disease. Although the precise causes of NCGS are unknown, it is known that gluten may nonetheless cause inflammation in those who have it.

Gluten may have an impact on intestinal permeability, sometimes known as "leaky gut." Gluten has the potential to elevate the synthesis of zonulin, a protein that controls the tight connections between intestinal lining cells in both NCGS and celiac disease. These tight junctions may become more permeable when zonulin levels increase, which might lead to the release of poisons, partly digested food particles, and other substances into the circulation. This may set off an immunological reaction that results in widespread inflammation. Chronic inflammation has the potential to aggravate several medical conditions over time, such as autoimmune illnesses, digestive difficulties, and even mental health concerns.

It takes more than simply staying away from apparent gluten sources like bread, pasta, and baked products to lead a gluten-free diet. Many processed meals and condiments include gluten. It's present, for instance, in processed meats, soups, salad dressings, and sauces. It's also often utilized in a variety of goods as a thickening or filler. It's important to carefully read labels since gluten may appear under a variety of names, including modified food starch, hydrolyzed vegetable protein, and malt. Cross-contamination, which may happen when gluten-free goods come into touch with gluten-containing foods during processing or preparation, is another issue to be mindful of. This may be avoided by using different cooking surfaces and utensils.

Thankfully, there are many wholesome gluten-free alternatives out there. Consider using grains and starches such as rice, quinoa, millet, buckwheat, and amaranth in place of items made from wheat. These grains include vital elements including fiber, protein, and vitamins, and are naturally gluten-free. Almond flour, coconut flour, and chickpea flour are examples of gluten-free flour that may be substituted in baking. Additionally, retailers provide a wide variety of breads, pastas, and snacks that are free of gluten and are manufactured with rice, maize, and potatoes.

Apart from these substitutes, concentrating on whole, raw foods may contribute to a wholesome and pleasurable gluten-free diet. Nutritious and naturally gluten-free include fruits, vegetables, lean proteins, nuts, seeds, and legumes. For instance, you may make delectable and well-balanced dinners with grilled meats or tofu, stir-fried vegetables, and fresh salads. Nuts, gluten-free granola, and fresh fruit are good snacks to keep your diet interesting and full.

Making the switch to a gluten-free diet can need some modifications, but it can be accomplished with proper preparation and knowledge. You may discover new favorites and keep a balanced diet by experimenting with various products and looking into gluten-free recipes. A nutritionist or dietitian may provide you with individualized advice and make sure your gluten-free diet satisfies all of your nutritional requirements.

You may lower inflammation and enhance your general health by learning about gluten sensitivity and how it affects inflammation and by leading a well-rounded gluten-free lifestyle. These tips may assist you in adjusting to a gluten-free lifestyle and leading a healthy one, regardless of whether you have celiac disease, non-celiac gluten sensitivity, or are just interested in learning more about the advantages of doing so.

The Benefits of Food Journaling

Food journals are an effective way to monitor your eating patterns, pinpoint triggers, and make well-informed dietary adjustments. You have the option of using classic paper diaries or digital applications, each with its unique benefits.

Advanced functions and convenience are provided by digital applications. With apps like MyFitnessPal, Cronometer, and Lose It!, you can quickly enter nutritional data, record your meals, and even scan barcodes. These applications often provide insightful data in the form of graphs and statistics, which facilitates the identification of patterns and trends in your eating habits. Many applications also include features that allow you to measure your water consumption, physical activity, and other health indicators, giving you a complete picture of your general health.

Paper journals, however, provide a more intimate touch. Writing by hand may promote more attentive eating and help you remain more involved in the activity. You may add your comments, observations, and doodling to personalize your writings in a paper notebook. It's also a fantastic choice if you'd rather work with your hands more or unplug from displays.

You need to record more than just what you eat in your food diary for it to be really useful. Provide specifics like the time of day you eat, the amount you consume, and how you're feeling both before and after. Taking note of your bodily sensations, such as headaches, bloating, or energy levels, may also provide insightful information. Keep track of your hydration levels and any physical activity you do, since these might affect your general health and the way your body reacts to certain meals. You may also examine how these factors interact with your diet and impact your overall well-being by monitoring your stress and sleep habits.

Using Diary Recordings to Determine Food Triggers

Identifying Correlations and Patterns: The capacity to detect trigger meals that may be generating unpleasant reactions or inflammatory responses is one of the key advantages of food journaling. You may begin to see trends and connections by keeping a regular journal of your eating habits and emotional state. For instance, you may notice a trend in your diary if you often have stomach problems after eating certain foods, like dairy or gluten. This might assist you in identifying certain meals or components that could be the source of the issue. Understanding how your symptoms connect to certain meals or food combinations may help you make informed decisions about which foods to change or avoid.

While keeping a diary might provide insightful information, consulting a nutritionist can improve the way you understand the findings. A nutritionist may assist you in reviewing your food journal, identifying possible trigger foods, and creating a customized strategy to deal with any dietary problems. They may also provide advice on how to choose a balanced diet, recommend substitute items or recipes, and assist you in putting any required dietary adjustments into practice. You may make sure that you're making well-informed choices regarding your diet and health and that your food journaling efforts are optimized by working with a specialist.

Keeping a food diary is an effective way to learn about your eating habits and how they affect your health. Whether you use a paper notebook or a digital tool, keeping a thorough diary of your food consumption, bodily sensations, and lifestyle choices can help you discover trigger foods and implement significant lifestyle adjustments to enhance your well-being. Your food diary may help you make educated dietary decisions and reach your health objectives by helping you identify trends and working with a nutritionist.

Diet's Impact on Male Hormones

Meals That Promote Optimal Testosterone Levels

Foods High in Zinc: Men's healthy testosterone levels depend on zinc, a vital element. It is important for the synthesis and control of testosterone. Oysters, which are especially high in zinc, as well as cattle, pigs, poultry, beans, nuts, and whole grains, are foods high in zinc. Ensuring appropriate intake via nutrition may assist promote hormonal balance and reproductive health since zinc deficiency has been associated with decreased testosterone levels and poor sperm quality. Including foods high in zinc in your diet may help improve your general health and immune system.

Healthy Cholesterol and Fats: Good fats are necessary to keep testosterone levels at their ideal levels. As a steroid hormone, testosterone is made from cholesterol. Thus, adding good fats to your diet may aid in the manufacturing of hormones. Olive oil, almonds, seeds, and avocados are good sources of healthful fats. Fatty fish like salmon, mackerel, and sardines are rich sources of omega-3 fatty acids, which are especially advantageous since they may lower inflammation and promote hormone balance. Maintaining appropriate testosterone levels may also be facilitated by consuming modest quantities of cholesterol from whole foods like eggs and lean meats. Consuming fat in moderation from a range of sources guarantees that your body gets the nourishment it needs to make hormones.

Dietary Components That Could Decrease Testosterone

Endocrine Disruptors in Food: Some ingredients in food can upset the balance of hormones, including testosterone, by acting as endocrine disruptors. Chemical additives used in processed foods, insecticides, and herbicides are common endocrine disruptors. These substances may cause endocrine system disruption by imitating or blocking natural hormones. For instance, phthalates and bisphenol A (BPA), which are included in a variety of food packaging materials, are known to alter hormone levels. Limiting exposure to these disruptors and promoting hormonal health may be achieved by selecting natural or less processed dietary items, cutting down on processed meals, and buying organic vegetables.

Impact of Obesity on Hormone Levels: The balance of hormones in the body, including testosterone levels, is significantly impacted by obesity. Having too much body fat, especially around the abdomen, might raise estrogen levels, which can work against testosterone. Additionally, a process known as aromatization allows fat cells to convert testosterone into estrogen. Reduced libido, exhaustion, and decreased muscle mass are some of the symptoms that might result from this imbalance and decreasing testosterone levels. Hormone management depends on maintaining a healthy weight via a balanced diet and frequent exercise. Consuming full meals like veggies, lean meats, and whole grains together with frequent exercise will maintain healthy testosterone levels and aid in weight management.

Maintaining optimum health requires an understanding of how nutrition affects male hormones. Hormone imbalances may be avoided by controlling obesity and being aware of endocrine disruptors, as well as by consuming foods high in zinc and healthy fats to maintain normal testosterone levels. You may enhance your general well-being and hormonal health by choosing foods wisely.

Making the First Dietary Adjustments

Setting practical objectives: Changing one's diet might be difficult, but it can go more smoothly if you create objectives that are both attainable and practical. Begin by pinpointing the precise areas you want to enhance, such as cutting down on processed meals, consuming more vegetables, or avoiding gluten. Divide these loftier objectives into more doable, smaller stages. If your objective is to eat more veggies, for instance, start with one meal a day and work your way up to one dish. Establishing short-term objectives, such as trying out one new nutritious meal per week, may boost your self-esteem and help you form enduring routines. It's crucial to exercise patience and flexibility and to make little, steady changes as opposed to trying to achieve perfection right away.

Packing and Preparing Meals: The secret to adopting dietary changes effectively is meal preparation and planning. Make a weekly food plan that includes breakfast, lunch, supper, and snacks. Based on your meal plan, make a shopping list to make sure you have everything you need. Meal prep in advance may save time and lessen the chance of selecting unhealthy selections. For hectic days, think about preparing meals in bulk and freezing them. Invest in high-quality containers to preserve the freshness of your food. Additionally, meal prep may be more fun and lead to the discovery of new favorites when you try out various recipes and cooking methods. Store a few basic dishes in your recipe book for those days when you just want something fast and healthy.

Overcoming Cravings: When attempting to alter one's diet, cravings may pose a serious challenge. The first step in controlling cravings is figuring out what sets them off, whether it is boredom, stress, or memories of certain foods. It's possible to sate urges by locating better options. Try some fruit or a little piece of dark chocolate, for instance, if you're craving sweets. By regulating blood sugar levels and prolonging feelings of fullness, eating balanced meals that include enough protein, fiber, and healthy fats may help minimize cravings. Finding healthy distractions from cravings, such as mindful eating and engaging in other activities, may also be beneficial tactics.

Out-of-Home Dining During an Anti-Inflammatory Diet: Eating out while following an anti-inflammatory diet might be difficult, but it is doable with little preparation. To start, go over menus in advance at restaurants to see what choices fit within your diet. A lot of restaurants may customize a meal or take unique requests, such as changing the ingredients or the recipe. Never be afraid to inquire about ingredients, cooking techniques, or other sources of sugar or gluten that may be disguised. Pick meals that are high in healthy fats, lean meats, and veggies. Choose steamed or grilled foods over fried or creamy ones when placing your order. To further prevent overindulging, think about splitting a meal or taking part in it at home.

There are numerous important tactics involved in diet-based inflammation reduction. Stress the benefits of eating a diet high in plant-based foods that are high in phytonutrients, which have anti-inflammatory qualities. Incorporate sources of good fats to help regulate hormones and lower inflammation, such as almonds, avocados, and fatty fish. Steer clear of hidden gluten sources and endocrine disruptors, cut down on processed meals, and practice good weight management. To promote general health, including a range of nutritious foods and well-balanced meals.

A comprehensive anti-inflammatory meal plan may facilitate the seamless integration of dietary modifications. Try a smoothie bowl with almond milk, chia seeds, berries, and spinach for breakfast. A filling and healthy lunch option is a quinoa salad with mixed veggies, chickpeas, and a lemon-tahini dressing. A grilled salmon fillet accompanied by steamed broccoli and roasted sweet potatoes might be the dinner option. Consuming fresh fruit, almonds, or hummus on veggie sticks for a snack might help you stay full and focused all day. It may be simpler to follow an anti-inflammatory diet and take pleasure in a variety of tasty meals if you include these meal ideas into your weekly schedule.

Making dietary adjustments calls for careful preparation and perseverance. You may establish a healthy and long-lasting eating routine by establishing sensible objectives, using efficient meal-planning techniques, and resolving frequent setbacks. Putting these dietary tips into practice and experimenting with different dishes can help you on your path to improved health and decreased inflammation.

4. TARGETED SUPPLEMENTATION

Essential Anti-Inflammatory Supplements

Omega-3 Fatty Acids

The anti-inflammatory benefits of omega-3 fatty acids, particularly eicosapentaenoic acid (EPA) and docosahexaenoic acid (DHA), are well recognized. By modifying the immune system and preventing the synthesis of substances that exacerbate inflammation, EPA contributes to the reduction of inflammation. On the other hand, DHA is vital for preserving the fluidity and functionality of cellular membranes, which is necessary for lowering inflammation and promoting brain health. Research has shown that consuming enough EPA and DHA may aid in the management of long-term inflammatory diseases such as depression, cardiovascular disease, and rheumatoid arthritis.

One may get omega-3 fatty acids from both plant- and animal-based sources. Fatty fish high in EPA and DHA, such as salmon, mackerel, and sardines, are examples of animal-based sources. Alpha-linolenic acid (ALA) is the main omega-3 found in flaxseeds, chia seeds, walnuts, and hemp seeds, for those who prefer plant-based choices. Although the body may convert ALA to EPA and DHA, this process is not very effective. As a result, those who eat a plant-based diet could think about taking supplements made of algae, which provide EPA and DHA directly and don't need conversion.

The amount of omega-3 supplements that are advised varies based on the health and dietary habits of the person. A typical daily dose for overall health is 500–1,000 mg of mixed EPA and DHA. Under the supervision of a medical professional, higher dosages could be advised for certain illnesses such as heart disease or inflammatory disorders. Although large dosages of omega-3 supplements may raise the risk of bleeding, particularly when coupled with anticoagulant drugs, they are usually thought to be safe. It is crucial to choose premium supplements devoid of toxins such as mercury.

Curcumin

Turmeric's major ingredient, curcumin, is well known for having strong antioxidant and anti-inflammatory qualities. Curcumin is not readily absorbed or used by the body, however, due to its low bioavailability. Supplements containing curcumin are sometimes mixed with piperine, which is included in black pepper, to boost absorption by up to 2,000%. To increase bioavailability, curcumin may also be combined with liposomes or lipids. Certain supplements use cutting-edge delivery methods, such as microencapsulation or nanoparticles, to improve absorption even more.

Certain medicines, such as antiplatelet agents, blood thinners, and treatments that alter liver enzymes, may interact with curcumin. These interactions may change how well the drugs work or raise the risk of bleeding. Before beginning curcumin supplements, it is crucial to speak with a healthcare professional, particularly if you are using prescription drugs or have a health issue that has to be closely monitored.

D-calcium

It has been shown that vitamin D affects inflammation and is essential for immune system control. Reduced vitamin D levels are linked to elevated inflammatory markers and an increased risk of long-term illnesses such as autoimmune disorders, cardiovascular disease, and arthritis. In addition to supporting general immunological function, vitamin D also serves to control the immune response and lower the generation of inflammatory cytokines.

You may get a blood test to measure your levels of 25(OH)D, or 25-hydroxyvitamin D, to find out whether you are deficient in vitamin D. Levels between 20 and 29 ng/mL may suggest insufficiency, while those below 20 ng/mL are often regarded as insufficient. A healthcare professional may suggest suitable supplements or lifestyle modifications to raise vitamin D levels based on the findings.

Age and health condition determine the recommended daily intake (RDA) for vitamin D; generally speaking, people should aim for 600–800 IU daily. For those with certain medical disorders or deficits, higher dosages can be required; nevertheless, a healthcare professional should be consulted before beginning any supplementation. Incorporating vitamin D-rich foods like egg yolks, dairy products with added fortification, and fatty fish into your diet is also advantageous. Additionally, getting sunshine exposure promotes the body's natural production of vitamin D.

More Important Supplements to Reduce Inflammation

Resveratrol: Known for its anti-inflammatory and antioxidant qualities, resveratrol is a polyphenol that may be found in red grapes, berries, and peanuts. By preventing the action of inflammatory enzymes and signaling pathways, it aids in the reduction of inflammation. The possible advantages of resveratrol for metabolic syndrome, neuroprotection, and cardiovascular health have also been investigated. The usual daily dosage range for supplements is 100–500 mg. Although resveratrol is typically safe, those on blood-thinning therapies should take it with care since it may interfere with these drugs.

Green Tea Extract: Packed full of polyphenols, especially epigallocatechin gallate (EGCG), green tea extract has potent anti-inflammatory and antioxidant properties. EGCG works by modifying inflammatory cytokines and pathways, which helps to lessen inflammation. Research indicates that green tea extract could be helpful for diseases including metabolic syndrome, cardiovascular disease, and arthritis. A typical daily intake of green tea extract is between 250 and 500 mg. Although it is typically well taken, certain drugs, such as blood thinners and stimulants, may interact with it.

Boswellia: Often referred to as frankincense, boswellia is a plant with strong anti-inflammatory qualities. It is beneficial for diseases like osteoarthritis and inflammatory bowel illness because it includes boswellic acids, which block inflammatory enzymes and pathways. Boswellia extract dosages typically consist of 300–500 mg taken two or three times a day. Although boswellia is typically harmless, some people may have stomach distress from it. Before using boswellia, like with any supplement, it is advisable to speak with your doctor, particularly if you are on any other drugs.

Alpha-Lipoic Acid: This antioxidant promotes the synthesis of cellular energy and lowers inflammation. Its potential advantages in situations including cardiovascular disease, age-related cognitive decline, and diabetic neuropathy have been examined. To improve the body's total antioxidant defense, alpha-lipoic acid may aid in the regeneration of other antioxidants. The usual range of recommended dosages is 300–600 mg daily. Although it is usually well taken, large dosages may interfere with diabetic treatments or create gastrointestinal problems.

Including these anti-inflammatory supplements in your routine may help control chronic inflammation and promote general health. It's crucial to choose premium supplements and speak with a medical professional to make sure they're suitable for your particular set of demands and ailments.

The Link Between Prebiotics and Probiotics

Supplements or dietary formulations known as synbiotics combine probiotics and prebiotics to improve gut health more successfully than each one does on its own. Prebiotics are indigestible fibers that function as food for probiotics, which are live beneficial bacteria that maintain a healthy gut microbiota. Synbiotics work by combining two helpful microorganisms (probiotics) and fostering and supporting the development of existing probiotics (prebiotics).

Easier immunological response, easier digestion, and increased nutritional absorption are among the advantages of using synbiotics. They may support the preservation and restoration of a healthy gut microbiome, which is essential for general well-being. Synbiotics may provide symptom alleviation and improve gut health for those with digestive diseases, such as inflammatory bowel disease (IBD) or irritable bowel syndrome (IBS). They could also enhance intestinal regularity, lessen inflammation, and boost a balanced immune system.

Specific probiotic strains combined with prebiotics that efficiently promote their development are known to form effective synbiotic combos. For example, inulin, a kind of prebiotic fiber, is often paired with Lactobacillus acidophilus, a typical probiotic strain. Combining Bifidobacterium bifidum with fructooligosaccharides (FOS) is another example. Combining these supplements has been shown to promote gut health by increasing probiotic colonization and survival in the intestines and encouraging the development of beneficial bacteria. Selecting synbiotics that include strains and prebiotics that have been scientifically demonstrated to act in harmony is crucial.

Selecting Beneficial Probiotic Supplements

Distinct probiotic strains have distinct health benefits, so they're not all made equal. Lactobacillus rhamnosus GG, for instance, is well recognized for its capacity to promote digestive health and lower the risk of gastrointestinal infections. Improved intestinal regularity and an enhanced immune system are two benefits of Bifidobacterium lactis. It's important to choose probiotic strains that have been studied and shown to work for your particular health issues when choosing a supplement. Seek supplements that provide comprehensive details on the strains they include as well as their shown advantages.

The term "colony-forming units," or CFUs, refers to the quantity of live bacteria in a probiotic supplement. Since the efficiency of a probiotic relies on the strain, the health issue being treated, and the bacteria's capacity to survive and enter the intestines, a larger CFU count does not always translate into improved efficacy. An intake of probiotic supplements typically contains 1 billion to 50 billion CFU. Lower CFU numbers may be enough for maintaining overall health, whereas higher counts may be necessary for treating certain medical conditions. To get the right CFU count for your requirements, refer to the product label's suggested dose and speak with a healthcare professional.

Probiotics that are shelf-stable vs those that need to be refrigerated: Probiotics may be either way around. Shelf-stable probiotics may be stored and traveled with ease since they retain their effectiveness even when left at room temperature. To maintain the vitality of the bacteria, they often use freeze-drying techniques. Conversely, cold storage is necessary for the efficacy of the live bacteria in refrigerated probiotics. These are often available at health food shops and are said to provide a better potency guarantee since the germs are preserved by the cold environment. Think about things like ease of storage and the manufacturer's suggestions for preserving potency when deciding between the two. If managed and preserved properly, both kinds may be useful.

Your gut health and general well-being may be improved by comprehending the link between probiotics and prebiotics, as well as the function of synbiotics and how to choose potent probiotic supplements. It is possible to promote a healthy microbiome, enhance digestion, and treat certain health issues by selecting the appropriate combinations and products.

Natural Probiotic Sources

Fermented Foods

Two of the most popular dairy-based probiotics are yogurt and kefir. Using certain bacterial cultures—usually Lactobacillus bulgaricus and Streptococcus thermophilus—milk is fermented to create yogurt. By enhancing digestion and regulating the intestinal microbiota, these advantageous microorganisms support gut health. Lactobacillus, Bifidobacterium, and helpful yeasts are among the wider variety of probiotic strains found in kefir, a fermented dairy beverage with a slightly sour flavor. Because of its wide range of microorganisms, kefir is well recognized for its ability to promote lactose digestion, boost immunological function, and improve digestion.

Buttermilk and certain cheeses, such as Gouda and cheddar, which also contain living cultures, are additional dairy-based probiotics. These goods may support a healthy gut microbiota and provide several health advantages, including as stronger immune systems and better nutritional absorption. To be sure you're receiving a product containing helpful bacteria, check for labels that state "live and active cultures" when selecting probiotics derived from dairy.

Kombucha, Sauerkraut, Kimchi (Non-Dairy Options): People who are lactose intolerant or who would rather eat plant-based foods have alternatives in the form of non-dairy probiotic sources. A symbiotic colony of yeast and bacteria is present in kombucha, a fermented tea (SCOBY). It may aid with detoxifying and digestion and provides a range of probiotic strains. Antioxidants and B vitamins are other ingredients in kombucha that support general health.

Fermented veggies like sauerkraut and kimchi are good sources of probiotics. Fermented cabbage is used to make sauerkraut, which also includes organisms like Lactobacillus plantarum. Kimchi, a traditional Korean fermented vegetable dish, contains several probiotic strains such as Lactobacillus and Leuconostoc, and is usually cooked with cabbage, radishes, and spices. Benefits from sauerkraut and kimchi include strengthened immunity, better gastrointestinal health, and higher vitamin and mineral intake.

Adding Probiotics to Your Diet

Daily Probiotic Food Suggestions: Including probiotics in your diet regularly doesn't have to be complicated or unpleasant. To begin, include a serving of kefir or yogurt in your daily breakfast or snack routine. Add fermented veggies, such as kimchi or sauerkraut, to sandwiches, salads, and side dishes. Use kombucha as a foundation for smoothies or enjoy it as a pleasant beverage. Try other fermented foods, like tempeh or miso, which are also full of good bacteria and can be used in a lot of different recipes.

Try to spread out your week's worth of probiotic-rich meals for a well-rounded strategy. To keep your gut microbiota in good shape, you must be consistent. To take advantage of the variety of probiotic strains that fermented foods provide, think about alternating between various kinds of fermented foods.

Home Fermentation Fundamentals: Maintaining fresh alternatives and savoring meals high in probiotics may be achieved via home fermentation. Start with easy dishes, such as yogurt or sauerkraut prepared from scratch. To make sauerkraut, shred the cabbage, add the salt, and pack it snugly into a jar. Leave it to ferment for a few days at room temperature. To keep yogurt at the right temperature for bacterial development, use a yogurt machine or a low-heat oven. To prevent contamination, strictly follow instructions and use clean containers and equipment.

Crafting kombucha, kefir, or even fermented pickles might be another way to experiment with home fermentation. To guarantee safety and efficacy, get starter cultures or SCOBYs from reliable suppliers and adhere to recommended fermentation procedures. You may develop customized probiotic meals and experiment with tastes at home using fermentation.

Supplement Safety and Considerations

Different interactions between supplements and drugs may change the way they work or raise the possibility of negative side effects. Garlic and fish oil, for instance, have been shown to thin blood. In combination with anticoagulant drugs such as warfarin, these supplements may increase the chance of bleeding. Comparably, St. John's Wort, which is often used to improve mood, might speed up how other drugs, such as birth control pills and some antidepressants, are metabolized, which may lessen their efficacy. Because St. John's Wort stimulates liver enzymes that expedite the breakdown of medicines, this interaction takes place.

Supplemental calcium may hinder the absorption of certain drugs, such as antibiotics or thyroid hormone replacements, reducing their effectiveness. Vitamin K may also have an impact on blood clotting processes, which is important to know if you're on anticoagulant medication. Moreover, medicines and herbal supplements like ginseng or ginkgo biloba may interact, changing the medication's effectiveness or safety. To prevent unforeseen effects, it is important to be aware of these interactions.

It is crucial to let your healthcare physician know about all of the supplements you use because of these possible interactions. This covers over-the-counter vitamins, minerals, herbs, and other nutritional supplements in addition to prescription drugs. Your healthcare practitioner may evaluate the safety and any interactions of your supplement regimen by using this information. They may recommend substitute supplements that won't conflict with your therapies or make the required changes to your medicine. This open line of contact reduces the possibility of side effects and guarantees that you get complete treatment. Your doctor can advise you on how to appropriately manage your supplement usage while taking into account your general health and any known medical issues.

Selecting premium supplements is essential to guaranteeing both their efficacy and safety. A method of confirming the quality of supplements is to seek independent testing and certifications. To make sure that supplements include the chemicals mentioned on the label and are free of contaminants, organizations like ConsumerLab, NSF International, and the United States Pharmacopeia (USP) do thorough studies. These certifications usually indicate that a product meets strict requirements for quality, potency, and purity. You may choose reputable and helpful supplements by looking for these endorsements.

Making educated decisions also requires skillfully reading supplement labels. Examine the supplement facts panel first, since it contains information on serving size, levels of active components, and their amounts. You may determine how much of a nutrient the supplement supplies about your daily requirements by understanding the percent daily values (%DV). In addition, go over the ingredient list to make sure there aren't any additives or allergies you may be concerned about. To verify the product's efficacy, make sure it is still within its expiry date. Information regarding the substances' sources, any interactions, and negative effects should all be included on labels. You may choose supplements that are both safe and appropriate for your requirements by carefully weighing these factors.

Tailored Supplements

The use of genetic testing in individualized health care—which includes choosing dietary supplements—is growing in importance. Our ability to digest and react to different foods and supplements might be influenced by our genetic composition. For example, some people may have genetic differences that impact how effectively they absorb certain minerals or how well they convert certain vitamins into their active forms. These genetic predispositions may be used to customize supplement selections to meet specific demands and improve health results.

Genetic testing, for instance, may determine if you have changes in genes that impact the metabolism of vitamin D. A larger dosage or a more bioavailable form of vitamin D may be beneficial for you if your findings show a decreased capacity to convert this vitamin into its active form. Comparably, genetic testing may provide information about your omega-3 fatty acid metabolism, which can help you choose the appropriate kind or quantity of fish oil supplement. You may improve the efficacy of your supplementing approach and make better judgments by incorporating genetic information into your supplement routine.

Working together with a healthcare professional is crucial when developing a customized supplement regimen. Your healthcare professional may provide advice on how to make supplement decisions based on the findings of your genetic test and can assist in interpreting the test results. To make sure that any supplements you take are suitable and safe, they may evaluate your general health, any current medical issues, and any drugs you are currently taking. It is especially crucial to seek expert advice when handling complicated medical conditions or using many supplements.

A healthcare professional may also assist you in creating a comprehensive supplement program that supports your overall health objectives. Based on your unique requirements, they may suggest certain supplements, track their efficacy, and change doses as needed. Frequent check-ups guarantee that your supplement regimen stays at its best even if your lifestyle or health circumstances change. Together, you may design a customized strategy that minimizes possible dangers and interactions and optimizes the benefits of supplementing.

We looked at several supplements in this chapter that have anti-inflammatory qualities. Flaxseed and fish oil include omega-3 fatty acids, which are well known for their capacity to lower inflammation and promote cardiovascular health. Turmeric's primary ingredient, curcumin, has strong anti-inflammatory properties, however, its bioavailability may be problematic. Supplementing with vitamin D, which is essential for immune system function and the control of inflammation, might be beneficial, particularly for deficient people. Moreover, several additional supplements have shown promise in lowering inflammation and promoting general health, including resveratrol, alpha-lipoic acid, green tea extract, and boswellia.

It's essential to adhere to recommendations for safe and efficient usage when adding supplements to your health routine. Before beginning any new supplement, always get advice from a healthcare professional, particularly if you have pre-existing medical issues or are already taking other drugs. Make sure the supplements you buy are safe and of high quality, having undergone independent testing. Read supplement labels carefully to ensure you are aware of the active components, doses, and any interactions. Personalized supplements may help you achieve your health objectives and make your routine more successful. It is based on genetic testing and expert advice.

5. MINDFUL ALCOHOL CONSUMPTION

Alcohol's Effects

Drinking alcohol causes inflammation in the body via several pathways that affect different organs and systems. Its part in hepatic inflammation is one important consequence. Alcohol is metabolized by the liver, and too much of it may exceed its capability, which can result in oxidative stress. Reactive oxygen species (ROS), which are released during alcohol metabolism and harm liver cells by inducing an inflammatory response, are the cause of this stress. A persistent inflammatory condition in the liver may be caused by fatty liver disease, alcoholic hepatitis, or even cirrhosis, which are all manifestations of liver inflammation.

Alcohol not only causes inflammation in the liver but also increases gut permeability, or "leaky gut," which negatively impacts gut health. Because alcohol damages the lining of the stomach, germs and poisons may cross the intestinal barrier and enter the circulation. As a result of the immune system's reaction to these foreign chemicals, this process causes systemic inflammation. This inflammatory reaction is made worse by the production of endotoxins, especially lipopolysaccharides (LPS) by gut bacteria. These endotoxins can enter the circulation, impacting other organs and causing broad inflammation.

Alcohol's inflammatory effects may be divided into short- and long-term effects, each having unique health implications. Drinking alcohol causes an acute inflammatory reaction in the short term. This includes brief elevations in immune cell activity and inflammatory markers, which may cause symptoms including warmth, swelling, and redness in the face. The symptoms of a hangover, which include general pain, electrolyte imbalances, and dehydration, might also be attributed to the acute inflammatory response.

Chronic alcohol use causes inflammation that becomes worse with time and stays longer. Long-term alcohol use raises oxidative stress and damages the liver continuously. Chronic inflammation has been linked to the development of dangerous medical disorders such as liver cirrhosis, liver fibrosis, and even liver cancer. Moreover, prolonged alcohol use has been related to systemic inflammation, which raises the risk of cardiovascular conditions including atherosclerosis and hypertension. Continuous endotoxin production from the stomach contributes to systemic inflammation, which worsens general health and raises the risk of chronic illnesses.

Moderate Alcohol Use

Health organizations often describe moderate alcohol intake as consuming alcohol in proportions that reduce health hazards while maintaining overall well-being. As per the recommendations issued by many health agencies, moderate drinking is often defined as one drink for women and two for men per day. 14 grams of pure alcohol, or about a 12-ounce beer, a 5-ounce glass of wine, or a 1.5-ounce shot of distilled spirits, is considered one normal drink.

The goal of these recommendations is to lower the risk of alcohol-related illnesses, such as liver disease, heart difficulties, and certain cancers. The goal is to provide individuals who want to drink a framework, not to promote alcohol use. Individuals may be able to prevent many of the negative consequences linked to increased alcohol consumption levels by abiding by these restrictions.

Differences based on Nation and Culture

It is essential to remember that national and cultural norms about moderation in alcohol use might differ. For example, depending on local beverage strengths and serving sizes, various nations may have varying definitions of what is considered a typical drink. Drinking habits and recommendations are influenced by cultural views on alcohol. Recommendations may be modified to account for variations in drinking habits or lower rates of alcohol use in other nations. Additionally, what is deemed moderate or acceptable in different civilizations might be influenced by cultural norms around alcohol drinking.

Health recommendations often strike a balance between promoting moderation in alcohol use and taking local customs and traditions into account. It is advantageous for people to evaluate their alcohol drinking patterns while taking cultural context and local regulations into account.

Differences in Alcohol Tolerance by Gender

Gender variations in biology have a big influence on alcohol tolerance and metabolism. Compared to males, women typically have a larger percentage of body fat and a smaller percentage of water. Women usually experience greater blood alcohol concentrations than males after ingesting the same quantity of alcohol because alcohol is dispersed in body fluids. The liver enzyme alcohol dehydrogenase, which breaks down alcohol, is also present in lesser concentrations in women. Due to this slower metabolism, the effects of alcohol may be felt more strongly and there is a greater chance of alcohol-related health problems.

Owing to these biological variations, women's health guidelines for alcohol intake are often more stringent. These variations in metabolism and the greater risk of negative effects explain the lower recommended consumption for women, up to one drink per day. Men are allowed to have up to two drinks a day due to their larger body water content and more effective metabolism of alcohol. These guidelines, which are based on gender, are meant to take into consideration physiological variations and lower the risk of alcohol-related health issues for both sexes.

Advantages of Cutting Back on Drinking

Enhanced Quality of Sleep

Alcohol significantly affects the architecture of sleep, often resulting in irregular sleep patterns. First, since alcohol has sedative properties, it may help you fall asleep. However, by decreasing the quantity of rapid eye movement (REM) sleep, which is essential for restorative sleep and cognitive function, it tends to disrupt the normal sleep cycle. Alcohol use may also result in fragmented sleep, which interrupts the continuity and quality of sleep by causing repeated awakenings throughout the night.

Eliminating alcohol may significantly improve the quality of your sleep. Longer durations of restorative sleep result from more regular and regulated sleep patterns without the sedative effects of alcohol. People often report higher overall sleep satisfaction, better REM sleep, and fewer nightly awakenings when their bodies adapt to decreased alcohol levels. Reducing alcohol intake has a major positive impact on sleep quality because it improves mood, improves alertness throughout the day, and improves cognitive performance.

Improved Liver Performance

Alcohol processing and metabolism are mostly carried out by the liver, and overindulgence in alcohol may cause damage to the liver, including cirrhosis, fatty liver disease, and alcoholic hepatitis. Reducing alcohol intake causes the liver to start healing and recovering. The degree of recovery is contingent upon the severity of the injury; nonetheless, significant progress is sometimes discernible in a matter of weeks to months. Reducing alcohol use may especially benefit fatty livers since the liver gradually regains normal function and inflammation levels drop.

Reduction in alcohol consumption is associated with improved liver function according to many indicators. Liver enzymes like aspartate aminotransferase (AST) and alanine aminotransferase (ALT), which are normally increased in instances of liver inflammation, are often shown to be normal in blood testing. Furthermore, symptoms including swelling, pain in the abdomen, and jaundice (yellowing of the skin and eyes) may go away. Improved liver function contributes to improved metabolic health overall by lowering the risk of major liver diseases and supporting improved detoxification procedures.

Improved Weight Control

Alcohol may negatively impact appetite and metabolism, which can lead to problems with weight control. It has no nutritional value and offers empty calories. Eating it might boost hunger and make bad eating decisions. Alcohol alters metabolic processes by interfering with the way fats and carbs are normally broken down, which often leads to an increase in fat accumulation. Alcohol may also affect how well the body controls hormones that stimulate hunger, which can result in a rise in caloric intake and weight gain.

Reducing alcohol consumption may result in large calorie reductions. For example, 150–200 calories may be found in a single serving of wine or beer, and having many drinks can soon mount up. People may save hundreds of calories a week by cutting down on or giving up alcohol, which can help them control their weight better. Additionally, consuming less alcohol might enhance nutritional selections since, while sober, individuals are probably going to choose better foods. Reduced calorie consumption and better eating practices work together to promote overall health and successful weight control.

Improvements in Cardiovascular Health

It is well-known that drinking too much alcohol raises blood pressure, which is a significant risk factor for cardiovascular illnesses. Blood vessel constriction brought on by alcohol use may raise blood pressure and resistance. People may assist control their blood pressure and minimize their risk of hypertension by consuming less alcohol. Better blood pressure management lowers the risk of heart disease and promotes general cardiovascular health.

Excessive alcohol intake is linked to a higher chance of arrhythmias, which are erratic heartbeats that may develop into life-threatening cardiac diseases like atrial fibrillation. Alcohol may cause irregular cardiac rhythms by interfering with the electrical impulses in the heart. Reducing alcohol consumption may improve cardiac rhythm stability and lower the chance of developing arrhythmias. People may so have fewer palpitation episodes and a lower chance of developing long-term cardiovascular problems.

Recognizing Problematic Drinking

Indications of Alcohol Addiction

Psychological and Physical Signs: Finding physical and psychological indicators of a problematic drinking connection is necessary to diagnose alcohol dependency. Increased tolerance, which occurs when a person has to drink more alcohol over time to have the same benefits, is one physical sign of dependency. Another obvious sign is withdrawal symptoms, which may include anxiety, trembling, sweating, nausea, and nausea when alcohol use is cut down or halted.

Addiction may also be indicated by physical health concerns such as liver damage, gastrointestinal disorders, or cardiovascular difficulties.

Strong alcohol cravings and an inability to reduce or regulate drinking despite a wish to do so are psychological traits of alcohol dependency. People who drink may find it difficult to balance their daily obligations and social activities, and they may spend a considerable amount of time either drinking or recuperating from its effects. Key psychological markers of dependency include increased attention to getting alcohol, disregard for personal or professional commitments, and persistence in drinking despite negative outcomes.

The **CAGE** Questionnaire: One often used screening test for possible alcohol abuse is the CAGE questionnaire. It comprises four questions used to evaluate drinking habits that may be problematic:

1. Cut down: Have you ever thought that you need to consume less alcohol?
2. Annoyed: Have you been irritated by remarks made by others about your drinking?
3. Guilty : When you drank, have you ever felt awful about it or guilty?
4. Eye-opener: To calm down or cure a hangover, have you ever drunk a drink first thing in the morning?

If you answer "yes" to two or more of these inquiries, you may be more likely to develop an alcohol habit. The CAGE questionnaire is an effective self-assessment tool that might encourage people to get further testing if necessary.

Tools for Self-Assessment

Online Screening Tests: To assist people in evaluating their drinking habits and possible dependency, a variety of online resources and screening tests are offered. These instruments often ask about the amount and frequency of alcohol consumed, how drinking affects day-to-day activities, and if withdrawal symptoms are present. Online tests that give a preliminary assessment of drinking habits, such as the Alcohol Use Disorders Identification Test (AUDIT) or the Brief Alcohol Screen, might be helpful for those who want to learn more about their relationship with alcohol.

When to Request a Professional Assessment: Self-assessment instruments are not a replacement for expert evaluation, even if they might provide insightful information. It's important to have a professional assessment if the findings of your self-evaluation point to problematic drinking or if there are any serious problems around alcohol use. Physicians, psychologists, and addiction specialists are examples of healthcare professionals who may give a thorough evaluation, a formal diagnosis if required, and a treatment plan customized to the patient's requirements. To successfully treat alcohol dependency and get the right resources and support for recovery, a professional assessment is essential.

The Effects of Excess Alcohol on Health

Liver Illness

Overindulgence in alcohol may cause a variety of liver illnesses, each of which advances through different phases. Fat buildup in liver cells is the hallmark of the first stage of fatty liver disease. Although there are often no symptoms at this point, if drinking persists, it might be an indication of more serious diseases. The next phase is known as alcoholic hepatitis. This inflammation of the liver may result in symptoms including nausea, vomiting, and jaundice. Alcoholic cirrhosis is a disorder where the liver becomes badly damaged and substantially impaired in function; it may develop from alcoholic hepatitis if treatment is not received. Complications from cirrhosis include an increased incidence of liver cancer, ascites (fluid buildup in the abdomen), and liver failure.

The degree of liver damage and a person's dedication to cutting down or quitting alcohol use determine how reversible the damage is. Cutting less on alcohol may often cure the effects of fatty liver disease. Early intervention and alcohol cessation may decrease inflammation and improve liver function in instances with alcoholic hepatitis. Cirrhosis, on the other hand, is an advanced form of liver damage that is mostly irreversible; while major liver damage from cirrhosis is often permanent, stopping alcohol use may stop further development and control symptoms.

Risk of Cancer Increasing

Long-term alcohol use has been associated with a higher risk of several cancers. Breast cancer is the most often linked cancer, especially in women, since alcohol may raise estrogen levels and encourage the development of tumors that are sensitive to hormones. Since cirrhosis and alcohol-induced liver damage are known risk factors, liver cancer is another major danger. Furthermore, cancers of the esophagus, mouth, throat, larynx, and colon are associated with alcohol consumption. The longer one drinks and the more alcohol they take in, the higher the danger.

Alcohol uses several methods to aid in the development of cancer. Its involvement in the production of acetaldehyde, a hazardous chemical that may harm proteins and DNA and cause mutations and cancer, is one important mechanism. Reactive oxygen species (ROS), which are also produced by alcohol, lead to further DNA damage and oxidative stress. Additionally, drinking may alter hormone levels and the metabolism of other carcinogens, increasing the risk of cancer. Alcohol is a strong risk factor for many types of cancer due to the combined effects of these pathways.

Inhibited Immune Response

Drinking too much alcohol weakens the immune system, making the body less able to fight off illnesses. Alcohol reduces the capacity of immune cells, such as neutrophils and macrophages, to react to infections. Moreover, it interferes with cytokine synthesis, which is essential for directing immunological responses. It is more difficult for the body to develop a strong defense against infections and recover from diseases when immune function is suppressed.

Alcohol usage impairs immunological function, which makes one more vulnerable to a variety of illnesses. Excessive alcohol use increases the risk of gastrointestinal and respiratory diseases, including TB and pneumonia. Alcohol weakens the digestive and respiratory tract mucosal barriers, which facilitates pathogen invasion and infection. Chronic alcohol use may also worsen the effects of illnesses and lengthen the time it takes to recover, which can further affect general health.

Alcohol-Free Substitutes

Recipes for Mojitos

Mocktails are non-alcoholic drinks made to provide classic cocktails' elegance and nuanced taste profile without the added alcohol. A delightful and spicy cocktail that combines fresh mint, lime, and sparkling water is the Virgin Mojito. An additional choice is a Cucumber Cooler, which is a refreshing and light drink made with cucumber slices, lemon juice, and a dash of tonic water. Ginger and Pomegranate Fizz is a tart, bubbly delight made with pomegranate juice, ginger ale, and a touch of lime. These mocktails are not only for those who don't drink alcohol; they are also tasty and entertaining substitutes for any kind of get-together.

Herbs and botanicals may add richness and depth to mocktails, making them more sophisticated. Drinks may be given distinctive tastes by adding fresh herbs like thyme, basil, and rosemary. For example, a Basil Lemonade incorporates basil leaves with the classic lemonade flavor. The Rosemary and Orange Spritzer is a fragrant and reviving mocktail made with rosemary syrup, fresh orange juice, and sparkling water. Aromatic and calming elements may also be added by botanicals like lavender and chamomile, which are ideal for blending into a sophisticated and calming beverage.

Social Techniques for Abstainers

While abstaining from alcohol while attending social occasions might be difficult, it is doable with the correct techniques. Bringing your non-alcoholic drink is one way to make sure you have something to drink and not have to depend on the few available alternatives. Another tactic is to concentrate on having talks and partaking in activities, such as games, debates, or other social gatherings, that do not revolve around drinking. Additionally, it might be beneficial to use assertiveness while defending your decision to abstain from alcohol, presenting it as a personal choice as opposed to a critique of other people's decisions.

The ability to sustain alcohol-free decisions is contingent upon having a supportive social network. Be in the company of people who appreciate your choice to give up drinking and who encourage you to make lifestyle adjustments. Interacting with communities or organizations that have similar objectives, including those that promote wellness and health or alcohol-free life, may provide accountability and support. Finding social gatherings and activities that don't center on drinking may also assist create a supportive and encouraging atmosphere where your decisions are valued.

Conscientious Consumption Habits

To practice mindful drinking, you should take time to enjoy every sip of your beverage. One technique is to take slow, little sips and focus on the scents, textures, and tastes of the beverage. Drinking mindfully may improve the experience and make it more pleasurable and fulfilling. In addition to allowing you to savor the sensory qualities of your drink, setting out devoted time to concentrate on it may also help quell the need to drink more fast or excessively.

Swapping out alcoholic drinks for water is another smart drinking technique. This strategy slows down the pace of alcohol intake in addition to keeping you hydrated. Water consumption in between alcoholic drinks may assist control total consumption, lessen the chance of overindulging, and lessen the chance of dehydration. This technique may also encourage a more balanced attitude to drink, enabling you to keep a healthy drinking pattern while still making use of the social components of alcohol intake.

The substantial effects of alcohol on inflammation and general health are discussed in this chapter. Drinking too much alcohol causes inflammation throughout the body, which raises the risk of cancer, damages the liver, and weakens the immune system. Alcohol-induced inflammation may proceed to more serious illnesses like cirrhosis and alcoholic hepatitis, although most often starts with fatty liver disease. Furthermore, there is ample evidence linking alcohol use to an increased risk of cancer, including malignancies of the breast, digestive system, and liver. Alcohol use is linked to cancer via oxidative stress, hormone abnormalities, and DNA damage.

Prolonged alcohol use also weakens the immune system, increasing a person's vulnerability to illnesses and decreasing their body's capacity to recuperate from sickness. Early intervention is critical for identifying problematic drinking practices using psychological and physical signs as well as instruments like the CAGE questionnaire. The negative health effects of binge drinking highlight the need to drink in proportion and with awareness to reduce inflammation and its related hazards.

6. RESTORATIVE SLEEP

Mostly via its roles in cellular repair and inflammatory management, sleep is essential for preserving general health. The body performs critical repair functions that are necessary for optimum performance when we sleep. The release of growth hormone, which mostly takes place during deep sleep, is a crucial component of this. Growth hormone aids in cellular renewal and repair, promoting the mending of muscles and tissues as well as the preservation of bone density. This hormone aids in the body's recovery from normal wear and tear by facilitating the repair of damaged cells and tissues.

Sleep is also essential for the activities that clean up cells. The glymphatic system in the brain eliminates waste materials that build up during waking hours. It functions best during sleep. This system lowers the risk of neurodegenerative illnesses and supports cognitive function by using cerebrospinal fluid to remove toxins and metabolic wastes from the brain.

Beyond the healing of cells, sleep is essential for controlling inflammation. The synthesis of cytokines—proteins involved in the immune response—is meticulously controlled while you sleep. Pro-inflammatory cytokines, which are involved in inflammatory reactions, and anti-inflammatory cytokines, which aid in reducing inflammation, are balanced by getting enough sleep. Maintaining this equilibrium is essential for avoiding chronic inflammation, which has been linked to several illnesses, including autoimmune diseases and heart disease.

There is a strong correlation between immunity and sleep. The immune system's capacity to efficiently combat infections and control inflammation is enhanced by getting enough sleep. On the other hand, insufficient sleep may upset this equilibrium, resulting in a rise in the synthesis of cytokines that promote inflammation and a compromised immune system. For this reason, keeping up appropriate sleep habits is crucial to controlling inflammation, boosting the immune system, and guaranteeing general health and well-being.

The Ideal Sleeping Time

Knowing the ideal length of sleep requires taking into account age-specific guidelines as well as the harmony between the amount and quality of sleep. Throughout life, sleep needs to alter dramatically in response to shifting biological and developmental demands.

Sleep is essential to a baby's and young child's development. The amount of sleep a newborn needs each day, which ranges from 14 to 17, steadily decreases as they become older. To maintain their cognitive and physical growth, school-aged children need around 9 to 11 hours, while toddlers and preschoolers typically need 11 to 14 hours. Because of their continuous development and changing hormones, adolescents have special demands that call for 8 to 10 hours of sleep per night to maintain their overall health and well-being.

The recommended sleep duration for adults is typically 7 to 9 hours each night. This length of time supports the preservation of ideal health, mental clarity, and emotional stability. Even if their sleep patterns may alter and they wake up more often and sleep for shorter periods, older folks still benefit from 7 to 8 hours of sleep every night to maintain their general health.

Individual differences in sleep needs are also significant. Although broad recommendations provide a foundation, individual variables including heredity, way of life, and general health may affect how much sleep a person requires. It's important to pay attention to one's own body and modify sleep patterns appropriately, since some people may do better with slightly less or more sleep than the suggested range.

Sleep quantity is not as important as sleep quality. There are numerous phases of sleep, such as light sleep, deep sleep, and REM (rapid eye movement) sleep, and each has a distinct purpose. While REM sleep is necessary for cognitive processes like remembering and learning, deep sleep is necessary for physical healing and development. For optimal rest and recuperation, the body must go through each of these phases of sleep in unbroken succession. Regardless of the overall quantity of sleep, disruptions like frequent awakenings or unfavorable sleeping conditions might counteract the restorative advantages.

Resolving Sleep Deficit

It is vital to acknowledge and tackle sleep debt to preserve general health and wellness. Over time, the accumulation of chronic sleep deprivation may lead to a variety of symptoms and indicators. One of the most prevalent signs is persistent fatigue when people often experience daytime tiredness even after receiving some sleep. This weariness is often accompanied by mood swings and anger, which makes it challenging to handle stress and have constructive interactions with others. Additionally, cognitive abilities deteriorate, resulting in issues with focus, memory, and judgment. Individuals may have difficulties with decreased attentiveness and delayed response times, which may affect how well they function in social and professional contexts. The effects of sleep debt are further highlighted by bodily symptoms like frequent yawning, a persistent feeling of being unrefreshed, and even physical health problems including decreased immune response and greater susceptibility to infection.

Sleep debt has a major impact on day-to-day functioning. Among the most noticeable side effects are emotional and cognitive deficits. People who don't get enough sleep typically have trouble concentrating, coming up with solutions, and making choices, which may lower their efficiency and productivity. The inability to regulate emotions results in elevated stress levels, heightened irritation, and challenges in managing social interactions. These side effects have the potential to exacerbate more significant health conditions down the road, including weight gain, cardiovascular disease, and a general decrease in one's capacity to handle stress in everyday life. Continuous sleep deprivation has a cumulative effect that may lower the quality of life and make it more difficult to carry out daily responsibilities.

Resetting sleep patterns strategically is necessary to address sleep debt. A prevalent misperception is that sleep deprivation may be counteracted by sleeping in on weekends. Weekend sleep-ins may help alleviate some of the exhaustion, but they don't completely offset the negative effects of chronic sleep deprivation on the body and mind. The body's internal clock may be thrown off by irregular sleep patterns, which includes weekend sleep catch-up. This makes it difficult to maintain a regular sleep schedule, which feeds the vicious cycle of sleep deprivation.

A more successful approach is to gradually modify the sleep routine. Maintaining regular sleep and wake time every day, including on the weekends, aids in the regulation of the body's circadian cycles and encourages higher-quality sleep. A more restorative sleep pattern may be easily adopted by gradually increasing the amount of time spent asleep by 15 to 30 minutes per night. It's critical to create a sleep-friendly atmosphere in addition to modifying sleep schedules. This entails making the most of the lighting and noise levels in the bedroom, keeping the temperature at a suitable level, and avoiding stimulants like coffee and electronic devices just before bed. Putting into practice a calming bedtime ritual, such as reading a book or having a warm bath, may help facilitate the shift to a more restful sleep. Patience and consistency are essential; gradual, continuous adjustments rather than abrupt cures lead to long-lasting gains in the quality of sleep and general health.

Lack of sleep and inflammation

The body's inflammatory processes are greatly impacted by sleep deprivation, resulting in a complicated interaction between insufficient sleep and elevated inflammation. Certain inflammatory markers are raised in the body during insufficient or disturbed sleep, which might result in a chronic inflammatory condition. Sleep deprivation has a special impact on important inflammatory cytokines including interleukin-6 (IL-6) and tumor necrosis factor-alpha (TNF-alpha). These cytokines are known to rise in concentration with inadequate sleep and are implicated in the inflammatory response. Increased TNF-alpha and IL-6 levels have the potential to aggravate inflammatory conditions and have a role in the emergence of chronic illnesses including diabetes and cardiovascular disease.

Lack of sleep also affects C-reactive protein (CRP) levels, which are a sign of systemic inflammation. Studies have shown that insufficient sleep is linked to elevated CRP levels, indicating heightened inflammation throughout the whole body. Increased CRP has been associated with heart disease, obesity, and metabolic syndrome, among other health problems. The correlation between CRP and sleep demonstrates how a prolonged inflammatory state may be exacerbated by chronic sleep deprivation, further impairing general health.

Inflammation and sleep deprivation are linked in a vicious cycle that may be hard to escape. Sleep patterns may be disturbed by inadequate sleep, which not only raises inflammatory indicators but also intensifies pre-existing inflammation. For instance, persistent inflammation may result in disorders like restless legs syndrome or sleep apnea, which can make it difficult to get deep, restorative sleep. An increasing number of health problems, such as mood disorders, chronic disease risk, and diminished cognitive function, might result from this recurring cycle of inadequate sleep and elevated inflammation.

Targeted therapies that improve sleep quality and manage inflammation are necessary to break this pattern. Creating a calm atmosphere before bed, adhering to a regular sleep schedule, and treating any underlying issues that can interfere with sleep are all helpful tactics. Stress-reduction tactics like mindfulness and relaxation training may lessen inflammation and enhance sleep. A balanced diet and frequent exercise are other components of a healthy lifestyle that may promote improved sleep and decreased inflammation. Through these therapies, people may address both inflammation and sleep, breaking the cycle and promoting general health and well-being.

Fostering Restful Sleep Practices

Establishing a sleep-friendly atmosphere is essential for attaining restful sleep and enhancing the general quality of sleep. Keeping the bedroom at the ideal temperature is essential to creating a sleep-friendly atmosphere. A colder temperature—generally between 60 and 67 degrees Fahrenheit or 15 and 19 degrees Celsius—can assist the body to recognize when it is time to go to sleep, therefore the bedroom should ideally be kept chilly. Furthermore, it's essential to regulate the illumination in the bedroom. Melatonin is a hormone that governs sleep, and it may be disrupted if bright lights or screens are exposed immediately before bed. Reducing computer time in the hour before bed and blocking out light with blackout curtains or an eye mask will increase melatonin synthesis and improve sleep.

Another crucial element in establishing a peaceful sleeping environment is noise reduction. Even little background noise might disrupt sleep, resulting in less restful or fragmented slumber. Using earplugs to block out distracting noises or white noise generators are two methods for minimizing noise. A calmer, more tranquil sleeping environment may also be achieved by making sure the bedroom is free of noise pollution sources like noisy appliances or road noises.

Cultivating good sleep habits also requires establishing a regular sleep routine. Consistent sleep patterns depend on the circadian rhythm, the body's internal clock, which is regulated by regular sleep-wake timings. Maintaining a regular bedtime and wake-up time, even on weekends, helps the body's natural circadian rhythm, which facilitates sound sleep and rejuvenation. Maintaining a regular sleep schedule helps the body's natural cycles and may guard against sleep problems like insomnia.

Resetting the circadian rhythm is a useful strategy for those who have trouble sleeping on irregular schedules. It might be helpful to gradually move the sleep pattern to a more desirable time by modifying sleep periods by 15 to 30 minutes every night. Furthermore, exposure to daylight throughout the day, especially in the morning, may support a healthy sleep-wake cycle and assist regulate the circadian rhythm. The body's shift to a more normal sleep pattern is further supported by avoiding stimulants like coffee and bright screens close to bedtime. People may enhance their general health and quality of sleep by setting up a sleep-friendly atmosphere and keeping to a regular sleep routine.

Your Sleep Improvement Toolkit

Enhancing the quality of sleep entails using a range of methods and instruments intended to augment relaxation and proficiently monitor sleep cycles.

Soothing Methods for Enhanced Sleep

Progressive muscle relaxation is a useful technique for improving sleep (PMR). This method entails methodically tensing and then releasing various muscle groups throughout the body. PMR eases physical and emotional stress by emphasizing the release of tension, which facilitates the descent into a peaceful state. Before going to bed, practicing PMR may help to relax the nervous system and encourage deeper, more rejuvenating sleep.

Sleep tales and guided visualization are two more beneficial relaxing methods. By using guided imagery, one may divert their attention from tension and worry by imagining a pleasant setting, such as a quiet forest or beach. Sleep tales provide calming narratives intended to calm the mind and facilitate the transition into sleep. They are often offered as audio recordings or applications. By fostering a calm and peaceful mental atmosphere, these techniques help facilitate falling and staying asleep.

Apps and Technology for Sleep Monitoring

Numerous techniques for monitoring and evaluating sleep patterns have been made possible by technology, providing information on the quality of sleep and possible areas for development. Various sleep metrics, such as sleep duration, sleep phases, and movement during sleep, are measured by sleep monitoring devices, such as wearable fitness trackers or specialist sleep monitors. These gadgets may provide insightful feedback on one's level of sleep quality and point out trends that could need modification.

However, there are benefits and drawbacks to utilizing sleep monitoring devices. Positively, these gadgets may provide users with comprehensive data on sleep patterns, assisting them in recognizing possible problems including inadequate sleep length or disturbances throughout the night. Making educated adjustments to sleeping patterns and raising the general quality of sleep may be greatly aided by this data. The drawbacks of relying too much on sleep monitors include the potential for anxiety related to sleep or a fixation with sleep metrics, both of which may impair the quality of sleep. Furthermore, it's important to use care when interpreting the data from sleep trackers since not all of them are equally reliable.

Trends rather than individual readings should be the main focus of sleep monitoring data analysis. To evaluate the general quality of your sleep and pinpoint potential causes of poor sleep, look for trends over time. For instance, it could be beneficial to change these behaviors if evidence consistently demonstrates that drinking coffee or partaking in stimulating activities before bedtime disrupts sleep. Working together with a medical professional or a sleep expert may also be beneficial in analyzing sleep data and creating a customized sleep improvement strategy.

People may improve their general well-being and quality of sleep by using progressive muscle relaxation, guided imagery, and other relaxation methods. They can also use sleep monitoring devices sparingly.

When to Speak with a Sleep Expert

When chronic sleep issues or symptoms point to a possible sleep disorder, seeing a sleep expert is a crucial first step. Knowing what to anticipate from a sleep study and identifying certain warning signals are crucial to determining whether to seek expert assistance.

Significant Causes of Sleep Disorders

A professional assessment is necessary to rule out sleep disorders, which may be indicated by specific symptoms. For example, the symptoms of sleep apnea include extreme daytime drowsiness, choking or gasping during sleep, loud snoring, and trouble remaining asleep. People who have sleep apnea may wake up throughout the night with recurrent breathing disruptions. This may cause sleep disturbances and several health problems, including hypertension, heart disease, and stroke.

Narcolepsy manifests as sudden, uncontrolled periods of daytime sleep, cataplexy (an abrupt loss of muscular tone brought on by intense emotions), and hallucinations or paralysis during sleep or wakefulness. If these symptoms are present regularly, it is imperative to obtain a diagnosis since they may severely affect daily functioning and quality of life.

Insomnia and other sleep disorders are characterized by trouble getting to sleep, remaining asleep, or waking up too early and not being able to go back to sleep. Prolonged sleeplessness may result in chronic exhaustion, agitation, and cognitive deficits, which can negatively affect general health and well-being. When to see a sleep expert may be determined by understanding these symptoms and how they may affect one's health.

A Sleep Study's Expectations

A polysomnography, also known as a sleep study, is a thorough assessment that's used to identify sleep problems. At-home and lab-based sleep research are the two main categories.

Key sleep metrics are measured in the comfort of one's own home with the use of portable monitoring equipment (also known as at-home sleep studies). These gadgets usually keep an eye on things like oxygen saturation, heart rate, and breathing patterns. Investigations conducted at home are more convenient and private than lab-based investigations, although they could provide less comprehensive data. They're often used in the diagnosis of ailments like sleep apnea.

Lab-based sleep studies may be carried out at a hospital or sleep clinic, offering a thorough understanding of sleep patterns via the use of a variety of metrics. Electrodes and sensors are applied to the body to record heart rate, respiration patterns, muscular activity, brain waves, and eye movements during lab-based research. A thorough examination of the phases of sleep and any potential disturbances is made possible by this configuration. A sleep lab's controlled setting aids in obtaining reliable data, however, it may not be the most pleasant place to spend the night.

Electroencephalography (EEG) measures the activity of the brain, Electrooculography (EOG) measures eye movements, and Electromyography (EMG) measures muscle activity during a sleep study. In addition, airflow sensors monitor breathing patterns, and pulse oximetry monitors blood oxygen levels. These informational pieces support the diagnosis of various sleep problems and direct recommended courses of action.

Options for Sleep Disorder Treatment

Various therapy strategies that are customized to the individual's requirements and the particular ailment are commonly used to address sleep disturbances. This is a summary of typical interventions, along with advantages and disadvantages.

Insomnia Cognitive Behavioral Therapy (CBT-I)

As a very successful treatment for chronic insomnia, cognitive behavioral therapy (CBT-I) focuses on altering the beliefs and actions that lead to sleep disturbances. Sleep education, sleep hygiene, sensory control, sleep restriction, and cognitive restructuring are some of the components of this treatment. Information on the significance of sleep and the variables affecting it is provided via sleep education. Establishing a sleep-friendly atmosphere is the fundamental goal of sleep hygiene, which includes sticking to a regular sleep schedule and limiting screen time before bed. By prohibiting some activities, such as reading or watching TV in bed, stimulus control assists patients in associating their beds with sleep. Sleep restriction shortens the amount of time spent awake in bed, and as efficiency increases, it progressively extends sleep duration. By addressing negative sleep-related beliefs, cognitive restructuring lowers anxiety and enhances the quality of sleep. Compared to medicine, studies have shown that CBT-I may dramatically increase the amount and quality of sleep, with long-lasting effects.

Phototherapy for Disorders of Circadian Rhythm

Disorders of the circadian rhythm, including seasonal affective disorder and delayed sleep phase syndrome, are treated with light treatment. Bright light exposure, often from a lightbox, is part of this treatment for a certain amount of time each day. The timing of light exposure is important because it may assist people with delayed sleep phase syndrome reset their internal clocks to an earlier time. Light exposure in the morning can do this. On the other hand, exposure to dusk light may be beneficial for those with advanced sleep phase disorders. By successfully resetting the circadian cycle to the intended sleep schedule, light therapy may enhance mood and sleep quality.

For temporary alleviation of sleep issues, over-the-counter (OTC) sleep medications such as antihistamines (doxylamine and diphenhydramine) are often utilized. Although they are widely accessible and simple to use, they often have negative consequences such as dry mouth, sleepiness throughout the day, and cognitive impairment. Furthermore, continued usage may cause their efficacy to decline and eventually result in dependency.

Prescription sleep aids are stronger and made expressly to treat sleep problems. Examples of these include benzodiazepines (like temazepam) and non-benzodiazepine hypnotics (like zolpidem). They have the potential to cause dependency or withdrawal symptoms, headaches, and dizziness, among other adverse effects, yet they may be useful in treating severe insomnia.

Because of these concerns, prescription drugs should only be used under a doctor's supervision and usually for a brief period.

Natural Supplements for Sleep

Natural sleep aids like valerian root and melatonin provide an alternative to pharmaceutical sleep aids. Melatonin, a hormone that controls the circadian rhythm, helps alleviate jet lag, sleep difficulties related to shift work, and delayed sleep phase syndrome. Supplementing with melatonin is typically regarded as safe, with few negative effects, such as headaches or vertigo. To guarantee efficacy, however, the dose and timing need to be well controlled.

Valerian root is a natural supplement that has long been used to enhance sleep quality and encourage relaxation. Although there is conflicting data supporting valerian's ability to shorten sleep duration and improve the quality of sleep, its long-term safety has not been well investigated. Drowsiness and stomach problems are possible adverse effects.

Adopting a multifaceted strategy that incorporates both practical measures and behavioral modifications is necessary to improve the quality of sleep. Establishing regular sleep schedules, improving the environment in which you sleep, and treating any underlying sleep problems with the right therapies are all important tactics for improving the quality of your sleep.

One of the main tactics is creating a sleeping-friendly atmosphere. This entails making the most out of the bedroom's features, such as keeping the temperature temperate, reducing exposure to light and noise, and making sure the sleeping surface is pleasant. Higher-quality mattresses and pillows, white noise generators, and blackout curtains may all make a big difference in how well you sleep. Additionally, by encouraging the creation of melatonin, limiting screen time and exposure to blue light before to bedtime helps the body's normal sleep-wake cycle.

Creating reliable sleep schedules is another essential tactic. Even on weekends, maintaining regular sleep and waking hours helps to control the circadian rhythm, which facilitates normal sleep and wake cycles. By lowering stress and anxiety, using relaxation methods like progressive muscle relaxation, guided imagery, or mindfulness meditation before bed may help improve the quality of your sleep.

It's crucial to speak with a sleep expert if you have persistent sleep issues or symptoms that point to a sleep disorder. Treatments for different types of sleep disturbances that work well include light therapy and cognitive behavioral therapy for insomnia (CBT-I). For those with circadian rhythm abnormalities, light treatment helps reset the internal clock, while CBT-I tackles the behavioral and cognitive components of insomnia. Making educated judgments on the usage of natural supplements like valerian root and melatonin, as well as sleep pharmaceuticals, requires an understanding of their advantages and disadvantages.

An action plan for healthier sleeping patterns is essential to successfully putting these tactics into practice. Begin by defining reasonable objectives, such as scheduling a regular sleep and wake-up time. Establish a calming nighttime routine gradually, which should include reducing stimulants such as coffee and large meals close to sleep. Adjust the sleeping environment as needed, paying particular attention to temperature, light, and noise levels. If you continue to have problems falling asleep, consult a doctor and think about having a sleep study done to identify and treat any underlying sleep disorders.

Through the implementation of these measures and adherence to a methodical action plan, people may notably raise the quality of their sleep, which will improve their general health and well-being.

7. BALANCED PHYSICAL ACTIVITY

Using Exercise as a Tool to Reduce Inflammation

Frequent exercise is one of the best ways to lower chronic inflammation, which is a major cause of many chronic illnesses. Through a variety of ways, exercise reduces pro-inflammatory markers and increases anti-inflammatory compounds in the body. These effects are shown in inflammatory processes.

Changes in inflammatory markers are one of the main ways exercise lowers inflammation. Muscles that are engaged in physical activity produce myokines, which are anti-inflammatory cytokines and other peptides. For example, it has been shown that interleukin-6 (IL-6) may suppress the production of tumor necrosis factor-alpha (TNF-α), a powerful pro-inflammatory cytokine, and that IL-6 is produced in significant quantities during exercise. Exercise also encourages the production of cytokines that reduce inflammation, such as IL-10 and adiponectin, which enhance metabolic health and reduce inflammation.

Grasp how exercise impacts inflammation requires a grasp of hormesis. The adaptive response of cells and organisms to mild stress, such as the stress brought on by physical activity, is referred to as hormesis. The brief stress that exercise causes to the body triggers several defense mechanisms that improve its capacity to handle stress in the future. To reduce chronic inflammation, this adaptive response involves repairing damaged tissues and upregulating antioxidant defenses. As a result, consistent exercise has a hormetic effect, making the body less susceptible to inflammatory stress.

Best Exercise Forms to Reduce Inflammation

It's crucial to participate in a variety of physical activities if you want to optimize the anti-inflammatory effects of exercise. While each kind of exercise has its benefits for lowering inflammation, a well-rounded regimen that includes weight training, aerobic exercise, and high-intensity interval training (HIIT) may be especially successful.

Benefits of Aerobic Exercise

The benefits of aerobic activity, including cycling, swimming, walking, and running, on reducing inflammation have been well-researched. Moderate to intense aerobic exercise improves cardiovascular health and enhances the body's capacity to control inflammation by raising respiration and heart rate. Studies have shown that consistent high-intensity physical activity may reduce levels of C-reactive protein (CRP), an indicator of systemic inflammation. Furthermore, aerobic exercise lowers oxidative stress and enhances endothelial function, both of which are linked to decreased levels of inflammation. Aim for at least 150 minutes of moderate-intensity or 75 minutes of vigorous-intensity aerobic exercise every week for the best anti-inflammatory effects.

Training for Resistance and Inflammation

Exercises that are performed against an external resistance, such as weights, resistance bands, or body weight, are referred to as resistance or strength training. This kind of exercise offers strong anti-inflammatory benefits in addition to increasing muscular growth and strength. Research has shown that resistance exercise may lower levels of inflammatory markers including CRP and TNF-α. Resistance training also contributes to improved body composition by lowering body fat and increasing muscle mass, both of which are linked to decreased systemic inflammation. For best results, a comprehensive resistance training regimen should work for all major muscle groups and be done at least twice or three times a week.

High-Intensity Interval Training (HIIT)

The goal of high-intensity interval training, or HIIT, is to alternate brief bursts of vigorous exercise with rest or lower-intensity intervals. The time-saving nature of HIIT and its ability to enhance metabolic and cardiovascular health have made it more popular. According to recent studies, HIIT may have anti-inflammatory properties as well. For instance, it has been shown that HIIT increases insulin sensitivity while lowering levels of inflammatory markers like CRP and IL-6. But it's crucial to approach HIIT cautiously, particularly for those who don't exercise much or who already have health issues. If HIIT intensity is not well controlled, it might initially lead to increased oxidative stress and inflammation. It is thus advised to begin with lower intensity intervals and work your way up to greater intensities.

To sum up, exercise is an effective way to lower inflammation and enhance general health. People may successfully manage and reduce chronic inflammation by learning how physical activity affects inflammatory processes and practicing a range of workouts. Regularly doing high-intensity interval training (HIIT), strength training, and aerobic exercise may all help increase the body's ability to withstand inflammation and improve long-term health.

Deciding on the Ideal Balance for Exercise

Maintaining general health and lowering inflammation need frequent physical exercise; nevertheless, striking the correct balance is critical to prevent overtraining and injury. It's important to recognize the warning symptoms of overtraining and learn how to adjust your workout regimen to your fitness level while allowing enough recuperation time. Overtraining may result in increased inflammation and a variety of other health problems.

Indications of Overexertion

When exercise volume and intensity surpass the body's capacity for recovery, overtraining takes place, resulting in symptoms that are both physiological and psychological. Overtraining may be physically manifested as chronic muscular pain, recurrent injuries, exhaustion, and a decrease in performance. Overtraining may also weaken the immune system and interfere with sleep habits, which increases susceptibility to sickness. Feelings of irritation, despair, and lack of enthusiasm to exercise are common psychological symptoms.

There is a noticeable inflammatory reaction to overtraining. Chronic inflammation may result from the body experiencing severe physical stress without sufficient healing time. Elevated levels of pro-inflammatory cytokines and other indicators, such as C-reactive protein (CRP), are indicative of this condition. Overtraining may cause persistent inflammation, which can worsen health and raise the risk of several illnesses, as opposed to the healthy, transient inflammation that comes with regular exercise.

Fitness Level-Based Exercise Selection

It's important to customize your workout routine to your current fitness level to prevent overtraining and optimize the advantages of exercise. Measure your physical strength, flexibility, cardiovascular endurance, and body composition to get a sense of your current level of fitness. A baseline may be established with the use of tools like fitness tests, health exams, or even expert evaluations to help create attainable and reasonable objectives.

In exercise training, gradual development is a fundamental concept. This entails gradually increasing the level of difficulty, length, and frequency of your exercises so that your body may strengthen and adapt without being overworked. It is advised for novices to begin with low- to moderate-intensity workouts and work their way up. More difficult routines may be added as fitness increases. To prevent damage and guarantee continued improvement, it's important to listen to your body and resist the impulse to push too hard too quickly.

Recovery and Rest Days Are Important

Every successful fitness regimen must include recovery. It lowers the chance of overtraining and injury by enabling the body to rebuild and strengthen itself in between exercises. Complete rest and active recovery are the two primary categories of recovery. Low-intensity exercises like strolling, mild yoga, or light stretching are examples of active recovery activities that may encourage blood flow and aid in muscle repair without adding to the load on the body. On the other side, complete rest entails abstaining from physical activity for whole days to give the body enough time to heal.

Including mobility and flexibility exercises in your program is another crucial component of healing. Static stretching and foam rolling are examples of mobility and flexibility exercises that may help preserve joint health, increase the range of motion, and avoid stiffness. These techniques improve overall movement quality and lower the chance of injury, which improves performance and long-term workout adherence.

Recognizing the symptoms of overtraining, adjusting your exercise regimen to your fitness level, and placing a high priority on recuperation are all part of striking the correct exercise balance.

Through attentive monitoring of your body's cues, you may modify your exercise regimen to circumvent overtraining and enjoy the manifold advantages of consistent physical exercise. This well-rounded strategy will improve your general well-being, help you maintain a healthy inflammatory response, and further your fitness quest.

Low-impact, home-based exercises

It's critical to find strategies to maintain your level of activity without overtaxing your body, particularly while managing inflammation. Low-impact, accessible exercises that can be done at home are a sensible alternative that has big advantages without needing expensive equipment or demanding schedules. These exercises may help reduce inflammation, increase physical fitness, and improve general well-being.

Yoga

Yoga is a very adaptable and easily accessible kind of physical activity that has anti-inflammatory properties. Various yoga forms, including Hatha, Vinyasa, and Yin, provide advantages that are specific to each practitioner's requirements and degree of fitness. Hatha yoga is appropriate for beginners and anyone looking for a peaceful practice since it emphasizes soft postures and deep breathing. While Yin yoga includes maintaining positions for lengthy periods and encouraging deep stretching and relaxation, Vinyasa yoga utilizes flowing movements and is somewhat more intensive.

Gentle twists, which facilitate digestion and detoxification, and restorative positions, such as Legs-Up-the-Wall and Child's Pose, which promote relaxation and stress reduction, are important poses for lowering inflammation. By lowering stress hormones, these positions help reduce inflammation. Frequent yoga practice may also decrease inflammation and promote improved general health by strengthening muscles, enhancing joint mobility, and improving flexibility.

Slow-motion Strength Training Activities

It's not necessary to use big weights or high-impact exercises for strength training. Without worsening inflammation, mild strength training activities with body weight or resistance bands may efficiently increase muscle mass and boost power. Beginners may work out at home with no equipment using bodyweight exercises like push-ups, lunges, and squats. By focusing on the main muscular groups, these workouts increase stability and strength.

An easy-to-transport and low-impact substitute for conventional weights is resistance bands. Exercises that offer resistance to develop muscle while being easy on the joints include banded rows, lateral band walks, and sitting band presses. Since resistance bands are available at several tension levels, as strength rises, the challenge may be gradually increased. This kind of exercise may assist in reducing inflammation, preserving muscle mass, and promoting metabolic health.

Beginning Walking Programs

One of the easiest and best low-impact workouts for beginners is walking. It is simple to include in everyday activities and doesn't need any specialized equipment. Increasing the length and intensity of walks progressively is the first step in a progressive walking regimen. As endurance increases, start with short, easy walks and progressively increase the duration.

A walking program's advantages may be increased by adding intervals and hills. Walking at a faster rate is alternated with a slower, recuperative pace during intervals. This method burns more calories and improves cardiovascular fitness. Including inclines in your workout—like hills or treadmill settings—increases its intensity and works multiple muscle areas, improving your overall fitness. Frequent walking can lower inflammation, assist with weight control, and enhance cardiovascular health.

Water Workouts

Exercises in the water provide a great low-impact workout that's particularly good for those with inflammatory or painful joints. Because of the buoyancy of water, motions are more painless and smoother. Without the burden of land-based activities, this setting enables a full-body workout that may enhance strength, flexibility, and cardiovascular fitness.

Swimming is a traditional water workout that strengthens every muscle in the body and improves cardiovascular health. Water aerobics is an enjoyable and efficient kind of exercise that includes doing aerobic movements in shallow water. Water's resistance is easy on the joints and aids in the development of strength and stamina. Other water activities include jogging or water walking, which have less of an effect than their land-based equivalents but provide comparable advantages.

Your health may be greatly improved by adding low-impact, at-home activities to your regimen. These include yoga, walking, lightweight training, and aquatic exercises. They also help to reduce inflammation and increase fitness. These exercises are appropriate for people of all fitness levels and those managing chronic inflammation since they are simple, flexible, and efficient. Finding something you like doing regularly can help you feel better overall and efficiently manage inflammation.

Special Considerations for Exercise

Incorporating exercise into a routine requires unique considerations to guarantee safety and efficacy, particularly for those with chronic diseases or restricted mobility. Exercise programs that are customized to meet individual requirements may help control symptoms, boost general health, and improve quality of life. An effective fitness routine requires knowing how to adjust activities and take drug interactions into account.

Working Out While Having Chronic Conditions

Because arthritis may cause stiffness and discomfort in the joints, exercise can be difficult. However, maintaining joint function and reducing the symptoms of arthritis need frequent physical exercise. Exercises that don't put too much strain on the joints, like yoga, cycling, and swimming, may assist preserve mobility and lessen discomfort. Muscles around the joints may be strengthened by strength training with modest weights or resistance bands, which improves support and lessens strain. It's crucial to begin cautiously, stretch gently, and stay away from high-impact activities that might make symptoms worse.

Exercise is essential for heart disease patients to manage their condition and enhance their cardiovascular health. To maintain safety, it is essential to adhere to certain criteria. Walking, swimming, and cycling are examples of aerobic workouts that are widely advised since they increase heart health and endurance. Patients should begin with brief exercises and progressively increase the time and intensity. It's critical to monitor heart rate and adhere to a safe range as prescribed by a healthcare professional. Strength training has its advantages as well, but it must be done carefully, with modest weights, and with an emphasis on technique.

Frequent exercise lowers the risk of problems associated with diabetes and helps regulate blood sugar levels. For those with diabetes, strength training and aerobic exercise are both advantageous. To avoid hypoglycemia, it's critical to check blood sugar levels before, during, and after exercise. It's a good idea to have fruit juice or glucose tablets on hand as a supply of quick-acting carbs. The primary elements of a healthy exercise program for treating diabetes include starting cautiously, continuing to exercise consistently, and drinking enough water.

Modifying Exercise Programs for Limited Mobility

Chair exercises are a useful approach for those with restricted mobility to remain active. These workouts might consist of stretching, aerobics, and even sitting weight training. Resistance bands, small dumbbells, or even your body weight may be used for a range of workouts that target various muscles. Chair-based workouts that increase strength and flexibility without forcing the user to stand include arm circles, leg lifts, and seated marching.

Making workout modifications to suit different skill levels guarantees that everyone may safely engage in physical activity. For instance, those who struggle with balance might do activities while providing support by holding onto a steady surface. Exercises that are modified to accommodate those with limited strength or flexibility, such as wall push-ups instead of floor push-ups, are a simple way to get started. To avoid injury and optimize advantages, it's critical to concentrate on using appropriate forms and make modifications as necessary.

Interactions Between Exercise and Medication

It's critical to comprehend the effects of certain drugs on the body's response to exercise to modify exercise regimens properly. For example, beta-blockers, which are often recommended for heart issues, may drop heart rate, making it difficult to determine the intensity of an activity based just on heart rate. Diuretics, which are used to treat high blood pressure, might make dehydration more likely, particularly while engaging in strenuous activity. It's critical to speak with a healthcare professional about any possible interactions between medications and exercise and to modify hydration and workout intensity as necessary.

Medication regimes might also affect when an individual exercises. For instance, to avoid hypoglycemia, diabetics who are insulin-dependent may need to schedule their exercise around their meals and insulin injections. Exercise during a time of day when one feels most awake if one is taking medicine that makes them drowsy. When planning an exercise, it might be helpful to know how drugs impact blood sugar, energy levels, and hydration. This can assist in maximizing safety and performance.

Including particular considerations in an exercise regimen guarantees that people with long-term illnesses or restricted mobility may participate in physical activity safely and efficiently. A customized fitness program that promotes health, controls symptoms and elevates quality of life may be made by modifying exercises, keeping an eye out for drug interactions, and speaking with medical professionals.

Optimizing Exercise's Effects

It's crucial to maximize several elements of your exercise regimen to fully benefit from exercise's anti-inflammatory properties. This includes not only how long and how often you exercise, but also how you eat afterward and how crucial it is to warm up and cool down correctly. These components are important for lowering inflammation and enhancing general health.

The Ideal Duration and Frequency of Exercise

To maximize the anti-inflammatory benefits of exercise, two factors are critical: its length and frequency. Studies indicate that at least 150 minutes of moderate-intensity aerobic exercise each week, distributed across many days, may effectively lower inflammatory markers. This equates to around 30 minutes of activity every day, five days a week, for most individuals. You may increase these advantages even more by including resistance and aerobic exercise in your regimen. Over time, chronic inflammation is reduced by regular physical exercise, which also helps control the production of anti-inflammatory cytokines.

But it's crucial to strike a balance between rest and recuperation and the volume and frequency of activity. Excessive training may counteract the benefits of exercise by causing inflammation to rise. Incorporating rest days into your regimen and paying attention to your body's needs are crucial for attaining sustained anti-inflammatory effects.

The Significance of Nutrition After Exercise

Nutrition after exercise is essential for lowering inflammation and promoting healing. Within 30 to 60 minutes after exercise, eating a balanced breakfast or snack that contains protein, healthy fats, and carbs will help restore glycogen levels, mend muscle damage, and lower inflammation. Protein aids in muscle growth and repair, while carbs replenish energy. Anti-inflammatory qualities found in healthy fats like those found in nuts, seeds, and avocados help the healing process even more.

You may increase the total anti-inflammatory benefit of your post-exercise meal by including anti-inflammatory foods like berries, turmeric, and green leafy vegetables in addition to macronutrients. Additionally, it's critical to maintain proper hydration since dehydration may worsen inflammation and impede healing. Maintaining a balanced inflammatory response and supporting appropriate body processes are two benefits of drinking plenty of water before, during, and after exercise.

The Significance of Adequate Warm-Up and Cool-Down

A workout regimen must include proper warm-up and cool-down practices, especially for lowering inflammation and avoiding injury. Warming up helps the body get ready for activity by raising blood flow, muscle temperature, and heart rate gradually. Dynamic stretches, mild aerobic workouts, and mobility drills that improve joint flexibility and lower the risk of strain may help accomplish this.

After working out, cooling down facilitates the body's return to rest, progressively reducing heart rate and assisting in the elimination of waste products from the metabolism. During the cool-down, static stretching may increase range of motion and release tense muscles. By lowering muscular discomfort and increasing circulation, self-myofascial release methods and foam rolling may further improve recuperation. Proper warm-up and cool-down techniques not only aid in injury prevention but also promote a quicker healing process, which lowers inflammation overall.

Tracking Development and Maintaining Motivation

Sustaining a regular exercise regimen and reaping the long-term anti-inflammatory effects need monitoring progress and being driven. A supportive fitness group, tracking inflammatory indicators, and setting reasonable training objectives may all assist in guaranteeing consistent dedication and improvement.

Tracking your progress and maintaining motivation requires setting reasonable, attainable workout objectives. Objectives have to be time-bound, relevant, quantifiable, achievable, and specified (SMART). For instance, setting goals like working out for 30 minutes five times a week or progressively lengthening and intensifying exercises provide precise time frames and benchmarks. As progress is achieved, breaking down more ambitious objectives into more doable, smaller ones may help keep you focused and give you a feeling of success.

Setting and reviewing objectives regularly in response to your body's reaction and development can help keep them fresh and challenging. Honoring little accomplishments and significant anniversaries along the path may increase drive and strengthen dedication to a healthy way of living.

Keeping an eye on inflammatory indicators might provide you with important information about how exercise is impacting your body. A routine physical examination with a medical professional may include testing for inflammatory markers including interleukin-6 (IL-6) and C-reactive protein (CRP). Monitoring these indicators over time will enable you to evaluate the success of your training program and make the required corrections.

Furthermore, subjective indications like increased vitality, less stiffness or discomfort, and general well-being might be used in addition to clinical tests. Monitoring these alterations may provide a comprehensive understanding of how exercise affects inflammation and overall health.

Motivation and commitment to a workout regimen may be considerably increased by becoming a member of an encouraging fitness community. Participating in online forums, joining neighborhood fitness organizations, or working out with loved ones may provide social support, accountability, and motivation. A feeling of camaraderie and dedication to fitness objectives may be fostered via participating in group activities, sharing experiences, and celebrating successes.

It is possible to increase the enjoyment and sustainability of exercise by starting or joining a fitness group that shares your interests and aspirations. Developing relationships with others who have similar health goals to your own may provide extra inspiration, encouragement, and a feeling of community, all of which can help you stick to an exercise schedule that is more efficient and reliable.

Optimizing workout length and frequency, paying attention to post-exercise nutrition, and implementing appropriate warm-up and cool-down routines are all necessary to maximize the anti-inflammatory effects of exercise. Setting reasonable goals, keeping an eye on inflammatory indicators, and participating in a motivating fitness environment may all be useful in tracking progress and achieving long-term health advantages.

The importance of exercise in reducing inflammation and enhancing general health was covered in this chapter. We discussed the several ways that physical activity—including weight training, aerobic exercise, and high-intensity interval training (HIIT)—can successfully lower inflammation. Exercise affects inflammatory indicators such as cytokines and C-reactive protein (CRP), which are important in controlling the inflammatory response of the body and lowering the risk of chronic inflammatory illnesses.

To maximize the anti-inflammatory effects of exercise, it is important to determine the ideal length and frequency of exercise. It is suggested that a balanced inflammatory response be maintained by participating in weight training in addition to 150 minutes of moderate-intensity aerobic activity each week. Maintaining a balance between exercise and rest periods is crucial to prevent overtraining, which may worsen inflammation and negate the benefits of physical activity.

Nutrition after exercise is also essential for lowering inflammation and promoting healing. Soon after working out, eating a well-balanced meal or snack high in protein, good fats, and carbs aids in muscle regeneration, inflammation reduction, and energy replenishment. Enhancing the effects of exercise and promoting general recovery may be achieved by incorporating anti-inflammatory foods and maintaining hydration.

The prevention of injuries and the promotion of efficient recovery depends heavily on following proper warm-up and cool-down regimens. An effective warm-up helps the body get ready for activity by raising muscle temperature and heart rate gradually, and a complete cool-down facilitates the body's return to its resting state. Stretching before exercise with dynamic movements and stretching afterward with static stretches improve flexibility and lessen pain in the muscles, facilitating a quicker recovery.

Maintaining a successful workout regimen requires evaluating inflammatory indicators and establishing reasonable goals to monitor improvement. Establishing realistic fitness goals and tracking your results regularly guarantee that your workout regimen stays in line with your overall health goals. You may stay inspired and dedicated to your workout regimen by creating a positive fitness community and acknowledging little victories.

The first step in creating a customized workout program is assessing your level of fitness at the moment and choosing regular, enjoyable activities. Include a range of workouts to target various facets of inflammation and fitness, such as resistance, flexibility, and aerobic conditioning. Adjust the plan to account for any unique medical needs or restrictions, and seek advice from medical professionals as necessary. Maintaining the efficacy and safety of your strategy requires regular reviews and adjustments depending on your body's input and development.

By putting these tactics into practice and making exercise the cornerstone of your anti-inflammatory regimen, you can improve your health tremendously, successfully control inflammation, and get the many advantages of regular exercise.

8. HOLISTIC SELF-CARE

A common misconception about self-care is that it only refers to luxuries or indulgent pursuits like spa days. True self-care, on the other hand, includes a comprehensive strategy for wellbeing that extends well beyond these surface-level considerations. To have a balanced and healthy existence entails attending to emotional, bodily, and spiritual requirements. Emotional self-care include mental health-promoting behaviors including stress management, counseling, and cultivating healthy connections. Maintaining body health via regular exercise, a balanced diet, and enough sleep is the emphasis of physical self-care. Taking care of one's inner life via spiritual self-care might include participating in activities that are consistent with one's values and beliefs or practicing mindfulness and meditation.

It's critical to see self-care as an essential health practice rather than only a luxury. It recognizes that resilience and general well-being depend on taking care of oneself. People may improve their quality of life, avoid burnout, and manage stress more effectively by incorporating self-care into their daily routines. This viewpoint promotes a proactive attitude to health, seeing self-care as an essential element of a well-rounded and satisfying existence, rather than a luxury or once-in-a-lifetime event.

Developing a Customized Self-Care Program

Creating a strategy that works for you requires evaluating your unique requirements and preferences to develop a tailored self-care regimen. Consider the aspects of your life where you could be putting your health last. Take into account things like your emotional and spiritual well-being, as well as your bodily health. This self-evaluation aids in pinpointing the precise self-care practices that will be most helpful to you. For instance, it might be helpful to include relaxation methods like yoga or meditation in your routine if you discover that stress is a big issue for you. A balanced diet and regular exercise may be crucial parts of your self-care regimen if maintaining your physical health is important to you.

Making deliberate decisions and allotting time for these activities in the middle of a hectic schedule is necessary for incorporating self-care into everyday life. You may make sure self-care activities become a regular part of your day by establishing a schedule that incorporates them. This may include setting aside time for workouts, making a menu, or practicing relaxation methods, and adhering to these schedules just as you would with any other significant endeavor. It's also beneficial to begin small and develop these habits gradually, modifying them as necessary to suit your tastes and way of life. Prioritizing self-care helps you live a more balanced and satisfying life by improving your general well-being and fostering resilience in the face of stress and adversity.

Inflammation of the System and Dental Health

The Link Between Mouth and Body

An important area of research that highlights how oral health issues may impact overall health is the relationship between systemic inflammation and oral health. The relationship between systemic inflammation and periodontal disease is among the most important. Chronic infection of the tissues that support the teeth and gums, known as periodontal disease, may cause inflammation not just locally but also throughout the body. The bacteria that cause periodontal disease can enter the circulation and cause inflammatory reactions. These reactions may lead to several systemic illnesses, including diabetes, rheumatoid arthritis, and heart disease. Systemic inflammation may be made worse by chronic inflammation resulting from periodontal disease, thus maintaining good dental health is essential.

The population of bacteria that live in the mouth, known as the oral microbiome, is also very important for general health. A well-balanced oral microbiome aids in the prevention of infections and illnesses and promotes a robust immune system. An excess of dangerous bacteria may result from disturbances in this equilibrium, which are often caused by poor nutrition or dental hygiene. This imbalance may affect systemic health and lead to inflammation. Sustaining a balanced diet and appropriate dental care promotes oral health as well as general well-being by preserving healthy oral microbiota.

Optimal Techniques for Dental Sanitization

Maintaining oral health and controlling inflammation requires practicing good dental hygiene. To get rid of food particles and plaque, which may cause gum disease and tooth decay, proper brushing and flossing practices are crucial. Brushing: All surfaces of the teeth and gums should be carefully cleaned twice a day using a soft-bristled toothbrush and fluoride toothpaste. To get rid of plaque and debris that a toothbrush cannot reach—the spaces between teeth and beneath the gum line—you should floss every day. Frequent dental examinations are also essential for expert cleaning and early identification of any problems.

Natural dental care techniques may enhance oral health and be used in addition to conventional ones. As an example, oil pulling using coconut oil is a custom that's said to lessen bad germs in the mouth and enhance gum health. Oral health may benefit from the anti-inflammatory and antibacterial qualities of herbal rinses, such as those that include sage or chamomile. But rather than taking the place of normal brushing and flossing, they should be used in addition to it.

By implementing these recommended techniques into everyday activities, systemic inflammation may be controlled and general health can be supported. Adhering to a strict oral hygiene regimen not only averts dental complications but also mitigates the likelihood of inflammatory ailments associated with oral health difficulties, thus promoting a more salubrious and harmonious lifestyle.

Therapeutic Massage Benefits

Various Massage Techniques for Inflammation

A variety of methods used in therapeutic massage may successfully decrease inflammation and improve general well-being. One of the most popular styles of massage is Swedish, which uses long, flowing strokes and light kneading to improve circulation and induce relaxation. This method supports the body's natural healing processes by reducing localized inflammation and promoting improved blood flow and muscle relaxation. Swedish massage may aid in reducing inflammation and promoting general physical comfort by reducing muscular tension and enhancing circulation.

Another helpful method is deep tissue massage, which is very useful for treating deeper layers of connective tissue and muscles as well as persistent muscular tension. More force and targeted manipulation on certain sore or uncomfortable regions are employed in this massage. Deep tissue massage can enhance mobility and decrease inflammation in specific regions by dissolving adhesions and scar tissue. This kind of massage is particularly helpful for those who have chronic stiffness or pain in their muscles because it increases the range of motion and facilitates healing.

The purpose of a lymphatic drainage massage is to precisely activate the lymphatic system, which is essential for eliminating waste products and extra fluid from the body. This soothing, rhythmic massage method aids in the reduction of edema and inflammation by promoting the passage of lymph fluid. People with illnesses that impair lymphatic flow or induce fluid retention may benefit most from it. In addition to helping the body's natural cleansing processes, lymphatic drainage massage is an effective way to reduce inflammation and enhance general health.

Tips for Self-Massage

Self-massage methods may be a useful supplement to professional massage therapy for the management of inflammation and the promotion of relaxation. Popular self-massage equipment includes massage balls and foam rollers, which allow you to apply pressure to certain body parts and relieve stress in your muscles. To reduce muscular tension and enhance blood flow, foam rolling, also known as self-myofascial release, is rolling a foam cylinder over the muscles. This method may assist decrease inflammation and promote recovery from everyday activities or exercise by releasing trigger points and increasing flexibility.

Massage balls may be used to target smaller or more focused regions of muscular tension. They are available in a variety of sizes and densities. Massage balls relieve localized discomfort by directly pressing on certain spots, improving circulation, and releasing knots. To relieve muscular discomfort and enhance general well-being, add these self-massage tools into your daily regimen.

Another useful self-massage method for reducing inflammation is acupressure. Acupressure points are places on the body where people may apply pressure to encourage the flow of energy and aid in healing. Acupressure points with specific benefits for pain and inflammation reduction provide a simple, all-natural means of assisting the body's inflammatory response. Acupressure may enhance other massage methods and promote better health and relaxation when included in a self-care regimen.

All things considered, including self- and therapeutic massage into a health regimen may be quite helpful for those who are controlling their inflammation. These techniques assist the body's natural healing processes, ease tense muscles, increase circulation, and enhance general well-being and relaxation.

Finding Toxins in the Environment

Household Common Toxins

Environmental pollutants are ubiquitous in many facets of contemporary life and often hide in our houses. Endocrine disruptors included in personal care items and indoor air pollution are common home poisons. Particulate matter and volatile organic compounds (VOCs) are examples of indoor air pollutants that may come from a variety of sources, such as paint, furniture, and cleaning supplies. These toxins may aggravate systemic inflammation and have a deleterious effect on respiratory health. For example, volatile organic compounds (VOCs) released by several home goods may result in poor indoor air quality, which is linked to several health problems, such as worsened respiratory and inflammatory disorders.

Hormone disruptors pose a serious threat as well. These substances, which may disrupt hormone function, are included in a wide range of personal care items, including lotions, shampoos, and makeup. Certain synthetic scents, phthalates, and parabens are examples of ingredients that can imitate or block hormones in the body, which may cause hormonal imbalances and associated health issues. Particularly over an extended period, exposure to these drugs may exacerbate systemic inflammation and other long-term health problems.

Means to Lower Exposure to Toxins

Reducing exposure to these environmental contaminants is essential for inflammation management and overall health maintenance. Making the switch to non-toxic home cleansers is one smart move. Harsh chemicals included in many traditional cleaning solutions have the potential to harm human health and increase indoor air pollution. Choosing eco-friendly or natural cleaning supplies lowers exposure to dangerous chemicals and promotes improved indoor air quality. Lemon juice, vinegar, and baking soda are a few examples of ingredients that work well for cleaning without the dangers that come with using professional cleaners.

Reducing exposure to toxins may also be achieved by filtering air and water. Water filters can eliminate impurities from tap water, including heavy metals, chlorine, and other dangerous materials. Similar to this, air purifiers with HEPA filters may aid in lowering allergens and particle matter in indoor air. The efficiency of these filtering systems in lowering the amount of pollutants present in the home environment is ensured by routine maintenance.

The "Body Burden" Concept"

The term "body burden" describes the total quantity of harmful substances that the body has acquired over time. This covers toxins found in the environment as well as those consumed via food, drink, and the air. Comprehending body load is crucial as it emphasizes the consequences of extended exposure to low concentrations of toxins and their ability to exacerbate chronic health problems, such as inflammation.

One important tactic for controlling body load is to encourage detoxification. Organs including the liver, kidneys, and intestines are involved in the body's natural detoxification processes, which aim to get rid of pollutants. The capacity of these organs to handle and eliminate pollutants may be improved by providing them with support from a nutritious diet, enough water, and frequent exercise. Including meals high in fiber and antioxidants may also help the body's natural detoxification processes and lower the body's total toxic burden.

Through the identification of prevalent environmental pollutants and the implementation of mitigation techniques, people may enhance their health management skills and bolster their body's capacity to metabolize and excrete toxins. In addition to enhancing general well-being, lowering body weight and encouraging a cleaner, healthier environment may have a big impact on controlling inflammation and enhancing medical results.

Skin Health and Protection

The skin is essential for shielding the body from irritants and inflammation from the outside world. Acting as a physical barrier to keep infections, poisons, and dangerous substances out of the body is one of its main purposes. The skin's microbiome, a varied collection of microorganisms that live on the skin's surface, supports the skin's barrier function. A balanced microbiome on the skin outcompetes pathogens and boosts immunity, preserving skin integrity and preventing inflammation. A disturbed microbiome, either from overuse of antimicrobial products or dietary imbalances, may weaken the skin's protective barrier and elevate inflammation.

The skin has a microbiome, but it also actively participates in immune function. Langerhans cells, among other specialized immune cells in the skin, aid in the detection and handling of possible dangers. To defend the body against wounds or infections, these cells can start inflammatory reactions. But if this reaction persists for an extended period or gets out of control, it may aggravate inflammatory skin diseases like psoriasis and eczema. Inflammation cannot be prevented or controlled unless the skin and its immune cells are kept in good condition.

Sensitive Skincare with Natural Ingredients

Selecting natural skin care products may help people with sensitive skin prevent irritation and reduce inflammation. Topical anti-inflammatory chemicals help maintain the skin's barrier function and calm sensitive skin. Known for their relaxing qualities, ingredients including calendula, chamomile, and aloe vera may help lessen redness and irritation. Furthermore, oils like jojoba and coconut oil aid in preserving the skin's natural barrier while offering hydrating properties.

Personalized skincare products devoid of irritating chemicals and harsh ingredients may be made with ease with homemade skincare recipes. With their anti-inflammatory qualities, simple recipes for homemade masks, scrubs, and moisturizers may use items like green tea, honey, and oats. For example, oats may provide mild exfoliation and hydration, while honey is well-known for its antimicrobial and calming properties. Making these products at home gives you more control over the materials you use and lets you customize skincare regimens to suit your requirements.

Inflammation and Sun Protection

To keep skin healthy and reduce inflammation, sun protection is essential. Overexposure to the sun may cause sunburn, early aging, and a higher chance of developing skin cancer, all of which exacerbate inflammation of the skin. Selecting the appropriate sunscreen is crucial for shielding the skin from damaging ultraviolet radiation. High SPF (sun protection factor) broad-spectrum sunscreens may help protect the skin from UVA and UVB radiation, lowering the risk of damage and irritation.

It's crucial to balance sun exposure for general health. Moderate sun exposure is important for the body to synthesize vitamin D, which promotes immune function and general health, even if too much sun may be hazardous. While allowing for restricted sun exposure, including sun protection measures—such as sunscreen use and protective clothing—can help preserve skin health and reduce irritation. People may enhance general well-being and strengthen their skin's natural defenses by combining these tactics.

Inflammatory Effects of Smoking

It is often known that smoking causes systemic inflammation, which affects many different parts of health. The introduction of hazardous substances into the body is the main way that smoking causes inflammation. More than 7,000 molecules, many of which are hazardous and capable of inducing inflammatory reactions, are found in tobacco smoke. These chemicals irritate the respiratory tract lining when breathed, which triggers oxidative stress and immune cell activation. Pro-inflammatory cytokines are released as a consequence of this activation, and these cytokines contribute to systemic chronic inflammation.

Smoking has an inflammatory impact outside of the lungs as well. Smoking aggravates systemic inflammation by negatively affecting many bodily systems. For instance, smoking increases the risk of endothelial dysfunction in the cardiovascular system, which affects blood vessel function and aids in the development of atherosclerosis, a disease marked by the accumulation of fatty deposits in the arteries. This vascular damage raises the risk of heart disease and exacerbates inflammation. Smoking also affects metabolic processes, increasing the risk of type 2 diabetes and insulin resistance. High levels of inflammation are linked to both of these illnesses.

Regardless of age, choosing to stop smoking has a major positive impact on one's health and significantly lowers inflammation. When someone quits smoking, their body goes through a healing process that might eventually lead to significant changes. The chronology of health gains after quitting smoking shows how amazing the body's healing power is. After only 20 minutes of cessation, blood pressure and heart rate return to normal. Lung function begins to recover and circulation improves in a few weeks.

Notable are the longer-term advantages. Compared to someone who smokes continuously, the risk of coronary heart disease is halved after a year. The risk of stroke drops to that of a non-smoker after five years. Compared to someone who keeps smoking, the risk of lung cancer is reduced after 10 years. In addition to these gains in health, there is a noticeable decrease in former smokers' levels of inflammatory indicators such as C-reactive protein (CRP). This decline illustrates the benefits of quitting on general health and shows a reduction in systemic inflammation. The advantages of quitting highlight the substantial health benefits that come with giving up smoking, demonstrating the possibility of recovery and enhanced well-being at any age.

Giving Up Smoking

Replacement Nicotine Options

The use of nicotine replacement therapy (NRT) is one of the best methods for stopping smoking. To lessen the desire to smoke and assist manage the symptoms of withdrawal, NRT delivers a regulated dosage of nicotine. There are several varieties of NRT accessible:

Patches: Nicotine patches help reduce cravings all day long by supplying a constant flow of nicotine via the skin. They may be worn for 16 to 24 hours and are available in different strengths.

Gum: Users may manage their nicotine dosage with this adaptable nicotine gum choice. Nicotine is released by chewing gum and is absorbed via the oral mucosa. It works very well for controlling impulsive cravings.

Lozenges: Slowly release nicotine after dissolving in the tongue. They function similarly to gum in that they provide an instant manner of satisfying cravings, but they are more covert and versatile.

Prescription drugs, in addition to over-the-counter NRT medicines, may help people stop smoking. By altering brain chemistry, drugs like bupropion (Zyban) and varenicline (Chantix) can lessen withdrawal symptoms and cravings for nicotine. When taken with additional measures, these drugs may dramatically increase the likelihood of successfully stopping.

Behavioral Methods

Behavioral techniques are essential for quitting smoking because they address the behavioral and psychological components of addiction. Approaches based on cognitive behavior (CBT) are very successful. CBT assists people in identifying and altering the mental processes and actions that lead to smoking. Identifying triggers, creating coping mechanisms, and establishing reasonable objectives are some techniques.

Moreover, practicing mindfulness might help you control your desires. Deep breathing, meditation, and progressive muscular relaxation are examples of mindfulness techniques that help people remain in the now and manage stress, both of which may lead to the desire to smoke. These methods may help one feel in control and at ease, which makes it simpler to withstand urges.

Systems of Support for Quitting

A robust support network is essential for a quit attempt to be effective. Options for group therapy provide a forum for discussing accomplishments, setbacks, and experiences with other people who are attempting to stop smoking. These meetings may provide support, useful guidance, and a feeling of unity.

Online forums and applications provide further assistance for smokers trying to give up. Apps for quitting smoking include tools for goal-setting, progress monitoring, and craving management. Additionally, a lot of them provide virtual health professional help and educational materials. Through advice and shared experiences, online communities and forums provide people access to a network of support and serve as a source of inspiration and responsibility.

To summarize, the use of behavioral methods, support networks, and nicotine replacement therapy may greatly increase the likelihood of successfully stopping smoking. These treatments provide a holistic approach to reducing nicotine dependency and attaining long-term success in quitting smoking because they target both the psychological and physical elements of addiction.

Activities & Hobbies that Reduce Stress

Creative Activities to Reduce Stress

One of the most effective ways to lower stress and encourage relaxation is to engage in creative hobbies. Pastimes like needlework, painting, knitting, or music may be good ways to let go of emotions and provide a mental retreat. By keeping the mind focused on the here and now and deflecting attention from worries, these activities promote happiness and a feeling of success. Making something may be very relaxing and fulfilling, offering a respite from the demands and routine of everyday life. Furthermore, studies indicate that engaging in creative activities might decrease cortisol levels, a major stress hormone, which in turn lessens overall stress and enhances feelings of well-being.

The Advantages of Outdoor Recreation

Another great way to reduce stress is to spend time outdoors. Hiking, gardening, or even just taking a stroll in a park may be quite relaxing activities. Spending time in nature has been connected to reduced stress hormone levels, happier moods, and sharper minds. The sounds of birds, the sight of greenery, and the feel of fresh air all provide a sensory experience that is calming to the mind and body while one is in the natural environment. Additionally, engaging in physical activity outside may enhance general health and lower stress levels by combining the healing powers of nature with the health advantages of exercise.

Everyday Mindfulness Practices

Daily routines that include mindfulness exercises may greatly lower stress and foster mental toughness. Being mindful entails giving the current moment your undivided attention. A calm and aware condition may be developed with the use of methods like gradual muscular relaxation, deep breathing exercises, and meditation. Regular mindfulness practice may improve stress management skills and reduce anxiety. It promotes a conscious attitude to day-to-day activities, which makes even tedious chores more interesting and less demanding. By keeping an eye on the present moment, mindfulness aids in ending the vicious cycle of tension and anxiety, encouraging a more tranquil and balanced state of mind.

Social Networks' Contribution to Inflammation

Having strong social ties is essential for controlling inflammation. Research has shown that those who have strong social support networks often have lower levels of inflammatory markers including interleukin-6 (IL-6) and C-reactive protein (CRP). Social connections improve mental health, lessen feelings of isolation, and provide emotional support—all of which may lessen the inflammatory effects of stress. Good connections help strengthen the immune system and regulate hormones, protecting the body from the damaging effects of stress. On the other hand, a greater risk of chronic illnesses and higher levels of inflammation are associated with social isolation and loneliness.

Although it takes work and intentionality to establish and maintain good relationships, there are many health advantages. Social relationships may be reinforced by regularly interacting with friends and family, taking part in neighborhood activities, and participating in group activities. Connecting with others who have similar interests and beliefs may be facilitated by volunteering or joining clubs and interest groups. Building connections requires effective communication skills, such as showing gratitude and actively listening. Making time for social engagements may also guarantee that these relationships stay solid and encouraging in the middle of hectic schedules.

We looked at a variety of holistic strategies for lowering inflammation in this chapter, stressing the need to take care of one's physical and mental health. Inflammation control and the promotion of general health are greatly influenced by the interconnection of our lifestyle decisions, which range from social interactions and stress management to nutrition and exercise.

Integrative methods of decreasing inflammation include taking part in stress-relieving pastimes and occupations including art, outdoor recreation, and mindfulness exercises. By reducing stress, these activities also decrease inflammatory indicators and promote mental and emotional well-being. While spending time in nature provides a sensory experience that soothes the mind and body, creative pursuits such as painting or performing music give an avenue for emotional expression and mental relaxation. Deep breathing exercises and other mindfulness techniques assist in interrupting the cycle of tension and anxiety by fostering a state of awareness and serenity.

We also emphasized the role that robust social ties have in reducing inflammation. Better mental health and reduced levels of inflammatory markers are linked to strong social support networks and positive interpersonal connections. Creating and sustaining wholesome connections through frequent social engagements, skillful communication, and community service may serve as a protective barrier against inflammation brought on by stress.

The process of incorporating these all-encompassing techniques into everyday life is creating a thorough self-care strategy. Achieving long-term health benefits requires evaluating each person's unique requirements for self-care and creating a customized regimen that includes social interactions, mindfulness exercises, and stress-relieving activities. Through purposeful decision-making to promote mental and physical health, people may successfully control inflammation and improve their overall quality of life.

Lowering inflammation requires a diverse strategy that takes into account social support, stress management, nutrition, and exercise. Individuals may cultivate a well-rounded and healthful lifestyle that eventually results in decreased inflammation and enhanced general well-being by adopting these holistic approaches and formulating an all-encompassing self-care regimen.

Conclusion

We have covered a wide range of tactics to reduce inflammation and advance holistic health in this book. The seven pillars of anti-inflammatory living—dietary choices, physical activity, stress reduction, good sleep hygiene, social interactions, environmental awareness, and tailored supplementation—have been discussed. Every pillar contributes significantly to the reduction of inflammation, and their interdependence emphasizes the need for a well-rounded and multimodal approach to health.

Including these techniques into your everyday routine is the first step in developing a customized anti-inflammatory regimen. Start by establishing reasonable expectations and objectives. Recognize that big changes need time and constant, deliberate work to manifest. Make tiny, doable changes at first, such as increasing your intake of plant-based meals, creating a regular exercise schedule, and making sleep a priority. Develop these habits gradually so that they become a vital part of your way of life. Customization is essential; what suits one person may not suit another, so adjust your strategy to fit your requirements and situation.

On this path, consistency and patience are crucial. The time it takes to observe noticeable benefits varies; for some, it may take a few weeks, while for others, it may take several months. Maintaining commitment and having faith in the process is crucial. Reward little accomplishments along the journey to keep yourself motivated. Recognizing that making lifestyle adjustments is a marathon, not a sprint, can help you maintain your focus on the long-term advantages as opposed to the short-term satisfaction.

It's essential to monitor your progress to modify your strategy as necessary. Keep a regular eye on inflammation levels using tools like wearables, blood testing, and symptom monitoring. Maintain a notebook to record any changes in your health and the effects of various tactics on your overall well-being. Don't be afraid to adjust your strategy if some of your tactics aren't producing the anticipated outcomes. Being adaptive and flexible is essential to developing a long-term anti-inflammatory lifestyle.

Research and therapy on inflammation have a bright future. New research and therapeutic approaches are constantly revealing more about the processes of inflammation and offering hope for improved outcomes. Novel anti-inflammatory chemicals, customized therapy, and genetic testing have the potential to completely transform the way we treat inflammation. Keeping up with these advancements will enable you to make well-informed choices about your health.

As we get to the end of this trip, you must give yourself the tools you need to take charge of your health. Mitigating acute symptoms is just one aspect of reducing inflammation; another is improving your general health and quality of life. Using anti-inflammatory tactics may have a cascading impact that increases mood, and energy, and lowers the chance of developing chronic illnesses. You are investing in a better, healthier future when you make deliberate decisions and dedicate yourself to a healthy lifestyle.

Recall that everyday decisions you make have the ability to change your health. Accept the trip with patience and an open mind. You are capable of attaining maximum health and minimizing inflammation, and each action you do will bring you one step closer to living a vibrant and well-being existence.

Printed in Great Britain
by Amazon